Microemulsions

Microemulsions

Edited by I. D. Robb

Unilever Research, Port Sunlight Laboratory
Bebington, Wirral, Merseyside, England

Plenum Press • New York and London

Library of Congress Cataloging in Publication Data

Main entry under title:

Microemulsions.

"Proceedings of a conference on the physical chemistry of microemulsions, orga-
nized on behalf of the Industrial Subcommittee of the Faraday Division of the Chemical
Society, and held September 15-16, in Cambridge, England"—Copyright p.
  Bibliography: p.
  Includes index.
  1. Emulsions—Congresses. I. Robb, I. D. II. Chemical Society (Great Britain). Faraday
Division. Industrial Subcommittee.
TP156.E6M5   660.2'94514   81-17766
ISBN 0-306-40834-1   AACR2

Proceedings of a conference on the Physical Chemistry of
Microemulsions, organized on behalf of the Industrial
Sub-Committee of the Faraday Division of the Chemical Society,
and held September 15-16, 1980, in Cambridge, England

© 1982 Plenum Press, New York
A Division of Plenum Publishing Corporation
233 Spring Street, New York, N.Y. 10013

PREFACE

The meeting on the Physical Chemistry of Microemulsions was organized on behalf of the Industrial Sub-Committee of the Faraday Division of The Chemical Society and held on September 15th and 16th, 1980 at Cambridge, U.K.

Microemulsions are attracting a wide interest not only in academic circles but also from industrial research and development units. From a fundamental point of view, these three component systems have a fascinating and complex array of structures that are providing a greater scope for investigation and debate than the simple surfact- ant-water micellar systems. The term microemulsion covers a broad range of molecular structures, unlike the more precisely understood terms applied in two component (surfactant-water) systems. A micro- emulsion is often thought of as being like a swollen micelle, though in practise the term covers systems ranging from those with clearly defined spherical structures to those possibly having no stable macroscopic interface at all. Many of these systems are represented in the contributions to this meeting. At the meeting there were lively and forthright discussions following the contributions. Whilst it is impossible to capture these accurately, something of their flavour is recorded in the Discussion section following each paper.

The best known industrial application for microemulsions is in tertiary oil recovery, where the low viscosities and interfacial ten- sions of the crude oil surfactant mixtures aid the removal of the oil from the porous rock formations. As experiments in the field are on such a large scale and sometimes require a few years to assess, a sound understanding of the basic physical chemistry of microemulsions is essential. Other applications are in the pharmaceutical, chemical manufacturing and detergent industries.

Thanks are due to Mrs. Linda Critchley for her rapid typing of the scientific manuscripts, without which these proceedings could not have been produced.

I. D. Robb
May 1981

v

CONTENTS

On the Phase Inversion in H_2O-Oil-Nonionic Surfactant
    Systems and Related Phenomena   1
    C.-U. Herrmann, G. Klar and M. Kahlweit

The Microemulsion Concept in Non-polar Surfactant
    Solutions   17
    H.-F. Eicke

Dynamic Light Scattering from Water Microemulsions
    in Organic Media   33
    J. D. Nicholson, J. V. Doherty and J. H. R. Clarke

Formation and Structure of Four-Component Systems
    Containing Polymeric Surfactants   49
    F. Candau and F. Ballet

Viscosity and Conductivity of Microemulsions   65
    K. E. Bennett, J. C. Hatfield, H. T. Davis,
    C. W. Macosko and L. E. Scriven

Structural and Solubilization Properties of Nonionic
    Surfactants. A Comparative Study of Two
    Homologous Series   85
    G. Mathis, J.-C. Ravey and M. Buzier

Dielectric Studies of a Nonionic Surfactant-Alkane-
    Water System at Low Water Content   103
    M. H. Boyle, M. P. McDonald, P. Rossi and R. M. Wood

On the Structure and Dynamics of Microemulsions. Self-
    Diffusion Studies   115
    B. Lindman, N. Kamenka, B. Brun and P. G. Nilsson

Phase Diagram and Interfacial Tensions of Brine-Dodecane-
    Pentanol-Sodium Octylbenzenesulfonate System   131
    A. M. Bellocq, J. Biais, P. Bothorel, D. Bourbon,
    B. Clin, P. Lalanne and B. Lemanceau

Alcohol Effects on Transitions in Liquid Crystalline
      Dispersions   143
   P. K. Kilpatrick, F. D. Blum, H. T. Davis,
   A. H. Falls, E. W. Kaler, W.G. Miller, J. E. Puig,
   L. E. Scriven, Y. Talmon and N. A. Woodbury

Connection Between Chemical Rate Coefficients and Two-Particle
      Correlation Functions in Aggregated Systems   173
   Sz. Vass

Fast Dynamic Processes in the Hydrocarbon Tail Region of
      Phospholipid Bilayers   185
   J. F. Holzwarth, W. Frisch and B. Gruenewald

Properties of High Emulsifier Content O/W Microemulsions
   R. A. Mackay.   207

Dynamic Processes in Water-in-Oil Microemulsions
   P. D. I. Fletcher, B. H. Robinson, F. Bermejo-Barrera,   221
   D. G. Oakenfull, J. C. Dove and D. C. Steytler

Ultrasonic Relaxation Studies of Microemulsions
   J. Lang, A. Djavanbakht and R. Zana   233

Index   257

ON THE PHASE INVERSION IN H_2O - OIL - NONIONIC SURFACTANT SYSTEMS

AND RELATED PHENOMENA

C.-U. Herrmann, G. Klar and M. Kahlweit

Max-Planck-Institut für Biophysikalische Chemie
Karl-Friedrich-Bonhoeffer-Institut
D-3400 Göttingen, FRG.

INTRODUCTION

In 1970 Saito and Shinoda[1] published a figure (Fig. 1) showing the effect of temperature on the volume fractions of the equilibrium phases of the ternary system

$$H_2O \text{ (A) - Cyclohexane (B) - } NP_{8.6} \text{ (C)}$$

where $NP_{8.6}$ stands for the surfactant polyoxyethylene (8.6) nonyl-phenylether. The figure also shows the effect of temperature on the interfacial tensions between these phases.

The system was composed of 47.5 wt % A, 47.5 wt % B and 5 wt % C. At room temperature one observes a lower phase rich in A and C and an upper phase rich in B. As the temperature is raised, the volume fraction of the lower phase increases at the expense of the upper phase. At $55^{\circ}C$ a third phase (a), rich in A, appears at the bottom of the vessel. Within a rather narrow temperature interval one thus observes three phases (a), (b) and (c) in equilibrium. As the temperature is further raised, phase (b) disappears, leaving only an upper phase, rich in B and C, and a lower phase, rich in A.

This phenomenon has been called phase inversion, and the temperature, at which it takes place, the phase inversion temperature (PIT).

In this paper we shall present an interpretation of this experiment on the basis of the effect of temperature on the phase diagram of the ternary system

$$H_2O \text{ (A) - Oil (B) - Nonionic Surfactant (C)}$$

1

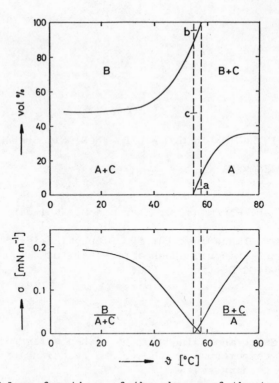

Fig. 1. (a) Volume fractions of the phases of the ternary system $H_2O - C_6H_{12} - NP_{8.6}$ versus temperature.
          (b) Interfacial tensions between the phases versus temperature (after (1)).

The considerations are based on the extensive studies of the phase diagrams of multicomponent systems at the beginning of this century [2].

In the second part it will be shown that in ternary systems of this type the effect of temperature is in many respects similar to that of an added inorganic electrolyte as fourth component.

Finally, we shall show that quaternary systems of the latter type may serve as model systems for multi-component systems of the type

$$H_2O - Oil(s) - Surfactant(s) - Salt(s)$$

which have been studied for the purpose of enhanced oil recovery.

The PHASE DIAGRAM A-B-C

The phase diagram of the ternary system A-B-C can be represented by an upright prism, the basis being the Gibbs phase triangle and the ordinate the temperature.

To discuss this phase diagram as function of temperature, we shall first consider the phase diagrams of the three binary systems A-B, A-C and B-C separately:

Fig. 2 shows the ternary phase diagram of the system A-B-C on a plane parallel to the basis at a temperature T close to the PIT. Also shown are the three binary phase diagrams, which form the outer planes of the prism.

i) A-B: water and oil are almost immiscible in the entire temperature range. Their miscibility gap will be denoted by γ.

ii) A-C: at low temperatures and low surfactant concentrations one finds a moleculardisperse solution of the surfactant in water. Above the cmc the excess of the surfactant molecules forms micelles. At high surfactant concentrations the solution becomes anisotropic: liquid crystals appear.

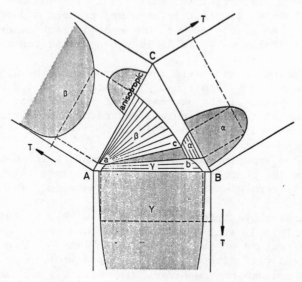

Fig. 2. Phase diagram of a ternary system A-B-C with three miscibility gaps at a given temperature (schematic). α,β and γ: miscibility gaps with tie-lines; shaded area: three-phase triangle with phases (a), (b) and (c).

As the temperature is raised, the anisotropic phases become
isotropic. At about the same temperature an upper miscibility gap
appears on the water rich side of the phase diagram, which widens with
rising temperature. This miscibility gap will be denoted by β.

The temperature at which water and surfactant separate into two
phases at a given surfactant concentration, is called cloud point.

The position and shape of this upper miscibility gap depends
strongly on the chemical nature of the surfactant: the higher the
oleophilicity - at a given hydrophilicity -, the lower the lower
critical temperature of the miscibility gap, and vice versa.

iii) B-C: Surfactants with low HLB-values (i.e. low hydrophilicity)
are completely miscible with oil. As the hydrophilicity is increased,
a lower miscibility gap appears on the oil rich side of the phase
diagram. This miscibility gap, which will be denoted by α, narrows
with rising temperature and finally disappears.

It should be noted, however, that in many cases this miscibility
gap does not appear right on the B-C plane of the prism, but only
after the addition of a little water.

All three miscibility gaps, the one between water and oil (γ),
the upper one between water and surfactant (β) and the lower one
between oil and surfactant (α) extend into the prism. If at a temperature T all three miscibility gaps are present and extend sufficiently deep into the prism so that they overlap each other, they form a
three-phase triangle a-b-c as it is shown in the centre of Fig. 2.

The unshaded areas in the three corners of the Gibbs triangle
represent homogeneous solutions. The three areas α, β and γ represent
two phase areas, i.e., the extensions of the three miscibility gaps
into the prism at this particular temperature. The straight lines in
these areas represent the tie-lines.

The shaded area in the centre represents a three-phase area.
Each solution the composition of which falls into this three-phase
triangle, will separate into the three phases (a), (b) and (c).

This three-phase triangle will exist within a limited temperature range only. It will appear at a temperature close to the (lower)
critical temperature of the binary miscibility gap β between water and
surfactant, and will disappear at a temperature close to the (upper)
critical temperature of the binary miscibility gap α between oil and
surfactant. Within this temperature range it will change its position
as well as its shape, depending on the effect of temperature on the
shapes of the three miscibility gaps in the ternary system.

The change of the position and shape of this three-phase region

within the prism has been nicely demonstrated by Shinoda and
Kunieda[3]. They determined the effect of temperature on the phase
diagram of the above system at a given surfactant concentration, varying the ratio between H_2O and oil (see their Fig.2). In other words:
they determined the number and nature of the phases, which appear, at
different temperatures, as one varies the composition of the solution
along a line parallel to the A-B side of the Gibbs triangle.

In accordance with our interpretation they found in the H_2O rich
region at low temperatures a homogeneous solution, which separates
into two phases at the cloud point. Between about 33 and 79 wt % oil
they found a lense-shaped three phase region (Fig. 3), the horizontal
distance between its boundaries giving the distance between the a-c
and the b-c side of the three-phase triangle at the corresponding
temperature and the corresponding surfactant concentration.

From Fig. 3 we conclude, e.g., that in this particular system
at 5 wt % $NP_{8.6}$ and $60^{\circ}C$ the three-phase triangle extends from 56 wt %
oil to 71 wt % oil in the Gibbs triangle.

PHASE INVERSION

Since in this particular system the binary miscibility gap β
widens with rising temperature, whereas the miscibility gap α narrows,
the three-phase triangle changes its shape in such a way, that the
length of its a-c side increases with rising temperature, whereas that
of its b-c side decreases. Consequently, point c moves from the water
rich side of the prism towards the oil rich side with rising temperature as it is shown schematically in Fig. 4. Let us now consider a

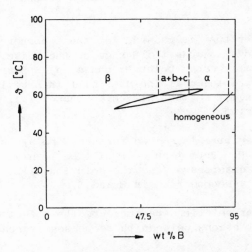

Fig. 3. Three-phase lense in the ternary system H_2O - C_6H_{12} - 5 wt %
$NP_{8.6}$ (after (3)).

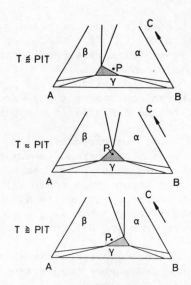

Fig. 4. Change of shape of the three-phase triangle with temperature (schematic). P: mean composition of solution.

solution, the composition of which is given by the coordinates of point P, and let us identify this solution with the one studied by Saito and Shinoda (Fig. 1). If at a temperature below the PIT the triangle has the shape as shown in Fig. 3a, P will be located in the miscibility gap α outside the three-phase triangle. Consequently, it will separate into a B-rich phase and a second phase rich in A and C.

As the temperature is raised, let the c corner of the three-phase triangle move towards the B edge of the prism. The b-c side will then eventually cross point P: phase (a) appears. Within a certain temperature interval, point P will then be located within the three-phase triangle, so that all three phases (a), (b) and (c) exist in equilibrium.

As the temperature is raised further, the a-c side will eventually cross point P. From then on P will be located in the miscibility gap β: phase (b) disappears, and the solution will separate into an A-rich phase and a second rich in B and C.

If this interpretation was correct, the effect of temperature on the interfacial tensions between these phases is readily understood.

Let us take the length of the tie-lines as a rough measure for the relative magnitude of the corresponding interfacial tension. As

P is approached by the b-c side of the three-phase triangle, the
length of the tie-lines of miscibility gap α will decrease. Consequently, the interfacial tension between the B-rich and the C-rich
phase will decrease increasingly rapidly until it reaches the value
corresponding to the interfacial tension between phase (b) and (c).
This value will be very low, since the b-c side of the three phase
triangle is the tie-line of the miscibility gap α closest to its
critical point.

As point P is crossed by the b-c side of the three-phase triangle,
the interface between phase (a) and (b) appears. Its tension will
first increase rapidly, as point P is approached and crossed by the
a-c side, to increase more slowly with increasing length of the tie-
lines of the miscibility gap β.

From the above considerations it follows that three-phase
triangles should not only exist in systems with "typical" detergents
as third component, but also with all amphiphilic substances, which
show a miscibility gap with both water and oil.

As an example we have studied the system (4)

H₂O (A) - Isooctane (B) - Benzyl alcohol (C)

in which each binary system shows a miscibility gap at room temperature. Consequently, one does find a three-phase triangle at room temperature. If the shape of this three-phase triangle is determined as
function of temperature (Fig. 5), one can easily find ternary solutions with an appropriate composition (P), which then show a phase
inversion with rising temperature similar to that found by Shinoda
and coworkers.

We thus conclude: i) A ternary system of the type

H₂O - Oil - Nonionic Surfactant

may show three miscibility gaps: one between H₂O and oil (γ), an
upper one between H₂O and surfactant (β), and a lower one between oil
and surfactant (α). The latter one, in particular, may not necessarily exist in a binary system oil - surfactant, but may appear only on
the addition of H₂O to the binary solution.
ii) If the three miscibility gaps overlap each other within a certain
temperature range, the ternary system shows a three-phase triangle
within its phase diagram, the (a) - (b) side of which does, in general
not fall onto the (A) - (B) side of the ternary diagram (Fig. 2).
The phase inversion observed in such systems can then be interpreted
as being the consequence of the fact, that this triangle moves across
the mean composition of the solution with rising temperature. Consequently, the so-called phase inversion temperature (PIT) is in fact a
temperature interval, in which this process takes place.

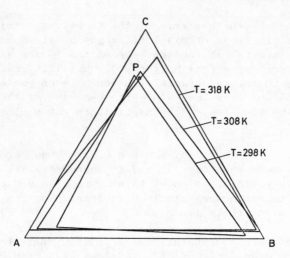

Fig. 5. Three-phase triangles in the ternary system H_2O – Isooctane – Benzyl alcohol as function of temperature; in wt % (after (4)).

iii) The position and shape of the three-phase region is mainly determined by the positions and shapes of the two miscibility gaps (α) and (β). Since for a given oil the miscibility gap (α) widens with increasing HLB-value, whereas gap (β) narrows with increasing HLB-value of the surfactant, the phase inversion temperature interval should rise with increasing HLB-value of the surfactant.

This prediction is supported by the findings of Shinoda and co-workers, who determined the three-phase lense (see Fig. 3) with $NP_{8.6}$(3), as well as with $NP_{9.7}$(5), both at 5 wt %. As one can see from a comparison of Fig. 2 in Ref.(3) with Fig. 1 in Ref. (5), the three-phase lense appears in the latter system at a temperature considerably higher than in the first system.

(iv) The application of "typical" detergents is not necessary for the existence of a three-phase triangle and a phase inversion, but can also be achieved by the application of "simple" amphiphilic substances like short chain alcohols. This suggests to study the simple systems as models for the more complicated ones, in particular with respect to the influence of the chemical nature of the surfactant on the position of the three-phase region as well as on the micro-structure of the different phases.

QUATERNARY SYSTEMS

In many ternary systems of this type the effect of temperature on the phase diagram is in many respects similar to the effect of an inorganic electrolyte as fourth component. As an example we consider the system

$$H_2O \text{ (A)} - \text{Benzene (B)} - \text{Ethylalcohol (C)} - (NH_4)_2SO_4 \text{ (D)}$$

which has been studied by Lang and Widom[6]. Again the alcohol plays
the role of a surfactant in this particular system.

The phase diagram of quaternary systems may be represented in a
tetrahedron, with the Gibbs triangle A-B-C as basis.

The ternary system A-B-C shows only one miscibility gap, namely,
the gap γ between water and benzene[7]. As salt is added, the two
other miscibility gaps α and β appear. Consequently, one does find
a three-phase triangle at a temperature as low as 21°C. In this case,
however, the plane of the triangle is tilted with respect to the basis,
phase (a), being rich in H₂O, having the highest salt concentration.

Fig. 6 shows the (vertical) projections of three of the nine
triangles, which were determined by the authors, onto the A-B-C basis.

For identification with the data published by Lang and Widom (see
their table I), the following list may be helpful:

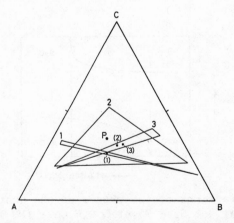

Fig. 6. Projections of some three-phase triangles in the system
H₂O-C₆H₆-C₂H₅OH-(NH₄)₂SO₄ at 21°C on the H₂O-C₆H₆-C₂H₅OH basis (after
(6)). The salt concentration increases in the order of the numbers.
The points in the centers of the triangles represent the mean composition of the corresponding solutions.

triangle 1 refers to mean $\left[(NH_4)_2SO_4 \right]$ = 7.61 wt %
triangle 2 $\left[(NH_4)_2SO_4 \right]$ = 9.76 wt %
triangle 3 $\left[(NH_4)_2SO_4 \right]$ = 10.55 wt %

Also shown on Fig. 6 are the projections of the corresponding mean composition of the solutions.

We note, that the projections published by the authors (see their Fig. 9) differ from ours. Their projections were obtained by projecting the triangles from the D-corner of the tetrahedron onto the A-B-C basis.

Although Lang and Widom did not keep the masses of A, B and C constant, to increase the mass of D only, their results may serve for the following considerations: If one considers a ternary solution A-B-C with the composition P and increases the salt concentration, P will first be located in the miscibility gap (γ) at zero salt concentration: the solution separates into a phase rich in A (and C), and a second one rich in B. As a sufficient amount of salt is added, the A-rich phase splits into two phases, one rich in A and D, the second one rich in C. As the salt concentration is increased, phase (a) moves towards the B corner. As the b-c side of the three-phase triangle crosses P^{*}, the solution separates into three phases: phase (a) appears. As the salt concentration is further increased, the a-c side of the triangle crosses P: phase (b) disappears. P is then located in miscibility gap β, the solution separating into a phase rich in A and D, and a second one rich in B and C.

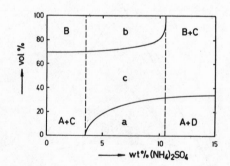

Fig. 7. Volume fractions of the phases of the quaternary system 35 wt % H_2O - 30 wt % C_6H_6 - 35 wt % C_2H_5OH - $(NH_4)_2SO_4$ versus salt concentration at $21^{\circ}C$.

*
With increasing salt concentration the projection of P moves slightly towards the center of the basis.

To confirm this prediction we have prepared a ternary solution composed of 35 wt % H_2O, 30 wt % benzene and 35 wt % ethanol and then added ammoniumsulfate at $21^{\circ}C$, keeping the masses of the three liquids constant and measuring the volume fractions of the phases as function of the salt concentration. The result is shown in Fig. 7.

As one can see, phase (a) appears at about 3.5 wt % salt, whereas phase (b) disappears at about 10.5 wt % salt, both values being in accord with the values interpolated from the change of shape of the three-phase triangles as determined by Lang and Widom.

For a more detailed discussion of such quaternary systems the reader is referred to the publications by Griffiths[8] and Lang, Lim and Widom[9].

TERTIARY OIL RECOVERY

Such quaternary systems may serve as models for the pseudo-quaternary systems studied for the purpose of enhanced oil recovery:

H_2O - Crude Oil - Surfactant - Salt

In practice the oil as well as the salt are mixtures of several natural components, whereas the surfactants used in tertiary oil recovery are in general mixtures of ionic and nonionic surfactants.

The phase diagram of such a pseudo-quaternary system is therefore more complicated than that of the simple quaternary system treated in the preceding section. Even if the salt was mainly NaCl, each component of the oil will show a different three-phase region, so that the observed phase behaviour will represent a superposition of many individual ones. The interpretation of the overall phase behaviour, however, should work alike.

As an example we consider the system

H_2O - Crude Oil - Surfactants - NaCl

which has been studied by Fleming et al[10]. The experiments were performed at $49^{\circ}C$, keeping the masses of H_2O, oil and surfactants constant and increasing the NaCl concentration. The result is shown in Fig. 8. The similarity between the phase behaviour of this pseudo-quaternary system and that of the true quaternary system shown in Fig. 7 is striking.

At low salt concentrations one observes two phases, one rich in H_2O and surfactant (labeled γ by the authors) and the second one rich in oil. In our interpretation these two phases correspond to the two equilibrium phases of miscibility gap α.

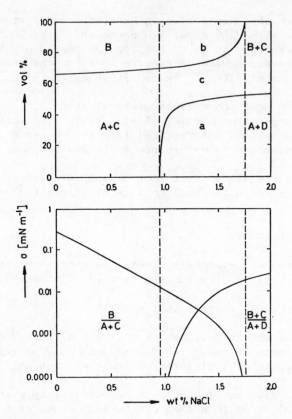

Fig. 8. (a) Volume fractions of the phases of the pseudoquaternary
system H_2O - oil - surfactant - NaCl versus NaCl concentration.
(b) Interfacial tensions between the phases versus NaCl concentration
(after (10)).

Between 0.95 and 1.8 wt % NaCl they observed three phases, a H_2O
rich phase appearing at 0.95 wt % and the oil rich phase disappearing
at 1.8 wt %. In our interpretation the b-c side of the three-phase
triangle crosses P at 0.95 wt % NaCl: phase (a) appears. As phase
(c) (labeled β by the authors) moves towards the B-corner, P is
crossed by the a-c side of the triangle at 1.8 wt % NaCl: phase (b)
disappears.

From now on P is located in miscibility gap β, separating into
a phase rich in H_2O (and NaCl) and a second one, rich in oil and
surfactant (labeled α by the authors).

The dependence of the corresponding interfacial tensions on salt concentration (Fig. 8b), too, is similar to their dependence on temperature in ternary systems (Fig. 1b). We thus conclude:

i) In many ternary systems of the type

H_2O - Oil - Nonionic Surfactant

the effect of temperature on the phase diagram is in many respects similar to that of an added electrolyte. Consequently, quaternary systems of the type

H_2O - Oil - Nonionic Surfactant - Salt

show a similar phase behaviour, if the salt concentration is varied instead of temperature.

ii) The position and shape of the three-phase region is mainly determined by the position and shapes of the miscibility gaps of the two ternary systems A-C-D and B-C-D.

iii) The application of "typical" detergents, in particular of ionic surfactants, is not necessary for the existence of a three-phase triangle and a phase inversion, but can also be achieved by the application of "simple" amphiphilic substances like short chain alcohols.

iv) Pseudo-quaternary systems of the type

H_2O - Crude Oil - Surfactants - Salt

show a similar phase behaviour with varying salt concentration as the true quaternary systems. This suggests to study the simple systems as models for the more complicated ones, in particular with respect to the influence of the chemical nature of the surfactants on the position of the three-phase region as well as on the microstructure of the different phases. Such an investigation may then yield qualitative recipes for the manipulation of the position of the three-phase region in a system with given oil and salt composition.

REFERENCES

1. H. Saito and K. Shinoda, J. Colloid Interface Sci., <u>32</u> 647 (1970).
2. F. A. H. Schreinemakers, in "Die Heterogenen Gleichgewichte", Ed. H. W. Roozeboom, Vol. III/2, Braunschweig (1913) G. Tammann, "Lehrbuch der Heterogenen Gleichgewichte", Braunschweig (1924).
3. K. Shinoda and H. Kunieda, J. Colloid Interface Sci. <u>42</u> 381 (1973).
4. U. Herrmann, to be published.

5. K. Shinoda, and H. Takeda, J. Colloid Interface Sci. $\underline{32}$ 642
    (1970).
6. J. C. Lang Jr., and B. Widom, Physica $\underline{81A}$ 190 (1975).
7. C.-U. Herrmann, U. Würz and M. Kahlweit, Ber. Bunsenges. Phys.
    Chem. $\underline{82}$ 560 (1978).
8. R. B. Griffiths, J. Chem. Phys., $\underline{60}$ 195 (1974).
9. J. C. Lang Jr., P. K. Lim and B. Widom, J. Phys. Chem., $\underline{80}$,
    1719 (1976).
10. P. D. Fleming, D. M. Sitton, J. E. Hessert, J. E. Vinatieri,
    D. F. Boneau, and R. E. Terry, SPE 7576 (1978).

DISCUSSION

Prof. F. Franks: Is not the P_{ij} concept an oversimplification? I
would expect surface behaviour to be much affected by the shape of
the surfactant molecule and the distribution of hydro- and oleophilic
residues, somewhat analogous to differences between block and random
copolymers composed of the same residues.

Prof. M. Kahlweit: We have chosen the polyglycolethers for our
further studies, because their shape as well as the distribution
between the groups remain congruent with changing i and j. If, however, one would compare the effect of the P_{ij}'s with other classes of
surfactants, one would certainly have to consider these differences.

Dr P. R. Rowland: Would you regard "P_{ij}" as analogous to "Equivalent
Carbon Number"?

Prof. M. Kahlweit: The term P_{ij} is equivalent to C_iE_j.

Prof. H. T. Davies: (i) The work of the University of Minnesota
group adds support to the position in this paper. We have published
work on alcohol-brine-hydrocarbon mixtures showing phase patterns
familiar to surfactant-brine-hydrocarbon systems. Furthermore we have
observed that the tension and volume uptake behaviour of the alcohol
systems is qualitatively to that of surfactant microemulsions. Thus
it appears that although the microstructure of microemulsion systems
may be special the pattern of their phase behaviour is not special
but is common to simpler solutions.

(ii) We have recently synthesized a series of ethoxylated hydrocarbons and have observed trends similar to the P_{ij} trends presented
here. The shape and height of the two phase dome is determined by
the number i of methyl groups and j of the ethoxy groups.

Prof. P. Stenius: Are your three component phase diagrams plotted on
a weight per cent or a mole fraction basis? If you plot them on a
mole fraction basis any formation of micellar solution and/or liquid
crystalline phases will be cramped into the surfactant corner and the
three phase triangle oil/water/liquid crystal will appear very large.

Prof. M. Kahlweit: The phase diagrams on our slides were plotted on the weight per cent scale.

Dr I. D. Robb: The PIT arises from the LCST and UCST on the H_2O oil and surfactant-oil axis respectively. As different anions have different effects (Hofmeister series) on these temperatures, does $(NH_4)_2SO_4$ have larger effects on the PIT than NaCl?

Prof. M. Kahlweit: Until now we have only studied the effect of different anions and anionic surfactants on the phase diagram H_2O-P_{ij}. Here the effect is very strong, in accord with the Hofmeister rule.

Prof. J. Th. G. Overbeek: Is there any information available on the interfacial tensions of the water-benzene-$(NH_4)_2SO_4$ system? In particular how low does the interfacial tension become in the three-phase region?

Prof. M. Kahlweit: Lang, Kim and Widon have measured the interfacial tensions between the three liquid phases (J. Phys. Chem. $\underline{80}$ 1719 (1976)). The values are in the order of one erg cm^{-2} and less, to be compared with 35 erg cm^{-2} between pure water and benzene.

THE MICROEMULSION CONCEPT IN NONPOLAR SURFACTANT SOLUTIONS

H.-F. Eicke

Physikalisch-Chemisches Institut der Universität Basel
Klingelbergstrasse 80
CH-4056 Basel (Switzerland)

It appears indispensable in discussing our present knowledge regarding the so-called microemulsions to point to the most problematic and unsatisfactory situation connected with the microemulsion notion. There does not exist as yet an operational definition of the microemulsion concept which is likewise useful for water-in-oil and oil-in-water systems. The main confusion seems to be due to the fact that microemulsions were originally defined purely phenomenologically, i.e. according to the observation that homogeneous, transparent, and low viscous solutions can be formed with considerable amounts of water or oil dispersed in the antagonistic continuous components in the presence of suitable surfactants and (eventual) co-surfactants.

If the most frequently encountered case is concerned, i.e. that the ternary system (H_2O, Oil, Surfactant) forms micelles in the limit x_{H_2O} or $x_{Oil} \rightarrow 0$, the question arises how to distinguish the microemulsive from the micellar state. In this connection it is important to realize that water-in-oil (W/O) and oil-in-water (O/W) "microemulsions" are not symmetrical from a physical point of view, although it might appear so from a phenomenological standpoint. Thus, it seems to be impossible, by any physical measurement, to detect a change in the properties of an oil-in-water emulsion in proceeding from an almost two-component to a three-component (Oil/surfactant/H_2O) system. The frequently used expression of "swollen" micelles certainly describes the situation satisfactorily in the latter system from a phenomenological standpoint. But - as already mentioned - there cannot be found any discontinuity in the physical properties of the system. Accordingly, the question as to whether we are concerned with a micellar solution or a so-called microemulsion cannot be answered from these experiments and may present a semantic problem.

17

It appears relatively easy to speculate why there should be a pronounced difference between water-in-oil and oil-in-water microemulsions. This has been done in a more quantitative way[1], but already qualitative considerations lead us to expect differences between these two emulsion types; micelles in aqueous solutions have always been described as being built up from an apolar core to which a "liquid" like structure has been ascribed. Generally, weak forces (dispersion forces) are then responsible for the interaction between the apolar tails of the micelles and the solubilized oil. Hydration interaction, i.e. mainly Coulombic forces, determine the state of the solubilized water-in-oil microemulsions. Hence, the physical situation is easily imagined to be rather different from that of the aqueous systems.

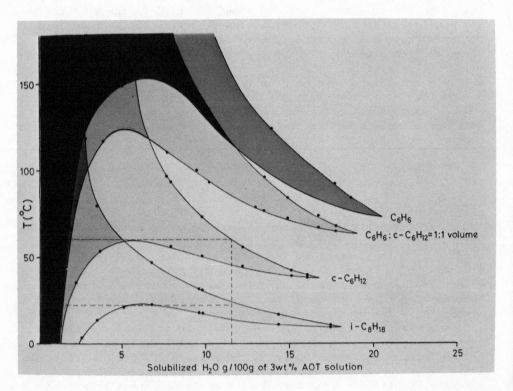

Fig. 1. Partial phase diagram of ternary H_2O/Aerosol OT/oil systems; the "tongue"-like regions are the so-called microemulsion domains[18].

We begin our considerations on microemulsions in non-polar media
with typical macroscopic measurements, i.e. a temperature versus the
amount of solubilized water-plot (Fig. 1) with different continuous
oil phases [1]. It appears noteworthy and not unexpected that the
micellar region (at low amounts of water) is indistinguishable with
respect to different hydrocarbon phases. This is certainly due to
the strong hydration interaction between water and the polar head
groups of the anionic surfactant (AOT) used in this example. With increasing amounts of solubilized water remarkable differences regarding
the positions of the transparent regions (= microemulsions) become
apparent. This can be interpreted thermodynamically to be due to different solubilities of the surfactant in these hydrocarbons ($i\text{-}C_8H_8 <$
$c\text{-}C_6H_{12} \lesssim C_6H_6$). This will be discussed later in more detail.

The optically transparent, low viscous, tongue-like regions are
equilibrium mixtures of inverted micelles, microdroplet-like particles
of water (or aqueous solutions) covered by a mono-molecular surfactant
layer, and also of lamellar liquid crystalline surfactant structures.
The latter may be considered as "nuclei" with respect to the experimentally proven phase inversion from W/O to O/W emulsive structures.
The state in between these two structures is frequently referred to
as a "bicontinuous state"[2,3]. The latter phenomena are to be observed close to the upper phase boundary, i.e. at the high temperature
limit of the microemulsion domain. At the lower phase boundary, the
above described pseudo-one-phase region separates into a two-phase
region containing the above mentioned microdroplets and free water.
The tips of the microemulsion domains are not at all well-defined.
They are accessible only via an extrapolation of the upper and lower
phase boundaries to larger amounts of solubilised water.

In order to obtain a more detailed insight into the physical chemistry of these systems, sophisticated physical techniques have to be
applied. To discuss the essential results in a consistent way it
appears reasonable to start with a short discussion of inverted micelles, since they not only contribute to the microemulsion region but
micellization and solubilization (= uptake of water by surfactant
structures) are also thermodynamical competitive processes[4]: the
temperature dependence of micellar sizes is a very suitable approach
in analyzing inverted micelles[5]. This has been done with a number
of alkali salts (including the ammonium ion) of di-2-ethylhexyl sulfosuccinates (Figs. 2 and 3). Quasi-elastic light scattering experiments can yield the temperature dependent hydrodynamic radii and the
polydispersity, i.e. $\mu_2/\bar{\Gamma}^2$ (μ_2 = second moment in the Pusey expansion
of the intensity autocorrelation function, $\bar{\Gamma} = \bar{D}q^2$ an average decay
constant with $\bar{D}$ the average diffusion coefficient of the particles and
$q = (4\pi n/\lambda_0)\sin \theta/2$, n = refractive index, θ = scattering angle and

[1]   Elaborated purification procedures may change shape and position
of the microemulsion domain. Nothing is changed, however, with respect to the arguments presented here.

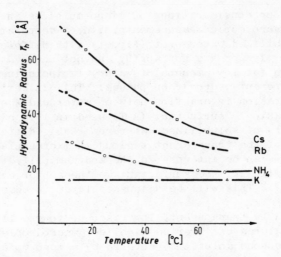

Fig. 2. Dependence of the mean hydrodynamic radii ($\overline{r}_h$) on the temperature for different alkali (including ammonium) salts of di-2-ethylhexyl sulfosuccinate.

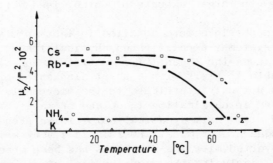

Fig. 3. Dependence of the variance of the particle size distribution (polydispersity) on temperature for alkali (including ammonium) salts of di-2-ethylhexyl sulfosuccinate.

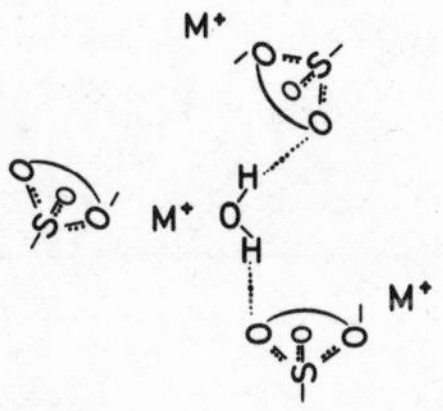

Fig. 4. Model for the formation of uni-valent sulfonate trimers at
low degree of hydration[6]

λ_0 = incident wavelength in vacuum) which is actually the variance
of the particle size distribution. Lithium and sodium (not shown in
the diagram) and potassium di-2-ethylhexyl sulfosuccinates exhibit a
remarkable independence of the hydrodynamic radii ($\bar{r}_h$) and polydispersities on temperature; the polydispersities of the Li-, Na-, and K-
salts are remarkably small and indistinguishable with the applied experimental method. An increasingly pronounced temperature dependence
is observed with ammonium, rubidium, and cesium salts. A tendency
towards less temperature dependent radii is, however, recognizable at
higher temperatures (Fig. 2.).

A model suggested by Zundel[6] to explain the properties of polystyrene sulfonate membranes appears also suitable to interpret the
experimentally observed properties of inverted micelles built up by
anionic surfactants of alkyl- or arylsulfonates (Fig. 4.). It is
assumed that one water molecule is attached to the counterion of a
surfactant (AOT) which is linked via two hydrogen bridges to other
sulfonate surfactant molecules, forming a kind of a network structure.
From this model it is to be expected that the stability of the aggregates (=micelles) depends on the hydration interaction between water
and the counterion and the strength of the hydrogen bridges. Both
effects, of course, will add up to the overall stability, however,
there exists an interesting possibility to judge the respective contribution of each effect by solubilizing deuterium oxide instead of
water. In this case the hydration interaction compared with water is
smaller (as is indicated by the lower heats of ionic hydration[7].
Due to the weaker attachment of the deuterium oxide molecule to the
counterion, the deuterium oxide solubilization results in a less
stable emulsive system compared to the analogous situation with
water[8].

The stability of network-like aggregates according to the above
model has been the subject of several calculations, e.g. [6,9]. Many
authors have stressed the importance of a field effect due to the
counterion on the proton in the hydrogen bridge (see Fig. 4) inducing

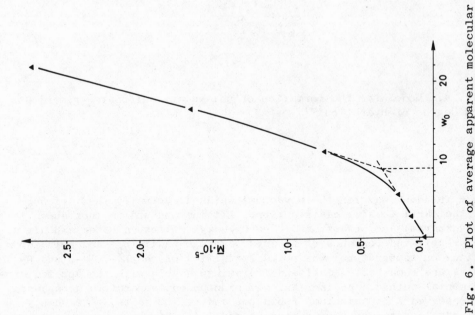

Fig. 6. Plot of average apparent molecular weight ($\overline{M}$) of micellar aggregate (AOT) against the amount of solubilized water $w_o = [H_2O]/[AOT]$, 298K

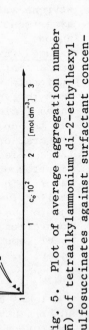

Fig. 5. Plot of average aggregation number ($\overline{n}$) of tetraalkylammonium di-2-ethylhexyl sulfosuccinates against surfactant concentration in benzene at 298 K[21]

a more symmetrical O - H ....O bridge with higher stability. From the results presented in this review it appears that the hydration inter- action with the counterion is essential if not dominating.

The weakening of the water-counterion interaction causes, for example, a significant decrease of the aggregate sizes (Fig. 5.) as is the case with tetra-alkyl ammonium ions.

If more water than the minimum amount necessary to form inverted micelles[10] is added to, say, an Aerosol OT (above the cmc)/isoctane solution, the micelles start to "swell". This initial state of the solubilization process could be followed by different experimental techniques. Fig. 6 exhibits the results of combined light-scattering and ultracentrifuge measurements[11]. It appears remarkable that the experimental points have to be represented by two curves: at small amounts of added water by a straight line, revealing a proportionality between the apparent average molecular weights of the aggregates and the amount of added water; at larger water content the curve rises non-linearly. The first part of the diagram has then to be interpre- ted as an uptake of water at constant number of aggregates, i.e. one observes a swelling process. Recent results from small angle X-ray scattering in non-polar Aerosol OT solutions with up to about 15 mol water per mol surfactant demonstrated that water is solubilized by swelling the aggregates[12]. The non-linear, steep branch of the plot is characteristic of a coalescence process which is accompanied by a decrease in the number of particles with a simultaneous increase in their sizes.

This swelling process is even better visualized if one considers the micelle to consist of some kind of network structure as may also be inferred from the model illustrated in Fig. 4. This picture is confirmed in addition by calculations of the average surface fraction of the water/hydrocarbon interface covered by one surfactant molecule as a function of the amount of solubilized water. The function is steeply increasing initially with small additions of water up to about $[H_2O]/[AOT] = w_o = 15$. Above this amount the value of the apparent surface fraction covered per surfactant stays approximately const- ant[11].

More detailed information on a molecular level is available from proton NMR spectroscopic measurements. Fig. 7 displays the dependence of three different proton chemical shifts in the water (D_2O)/Aerosol OT/isoctane system for variable amounts of $H_2O(D_2O)$ considering first the water proton, it is seen that with small amounts of added water, i.e. $w_o < 10$, an increasing up-field shift is observed as a direct indication of the disruption of the bulk liquid-like water structure at the interface and the formation of relatively rigid association structures through strong hydrogen bonding with the polar groups of the Aerosol OT. Within the range $10 \lesssim w_o \lesssim 20$ water molecules are partly free within the aggregates. The water protons experience, how-

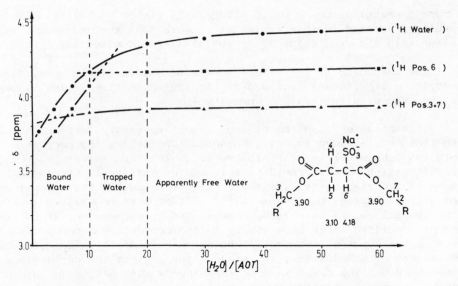

Fig. 7. Dependence of chemical shifts (δ) of three different protons against the amount of solubilized water $w_o = [H_2O]/[AOT]$ in the system: H_2O/Aerosol OT/i-C_8H_8, 298K.

ever, a rapid exchange between strongly and less bound water. This water-type may, therefore, be called "trapped" water. With still larger amounts of water the latter adopts the character of apparently free water, of course containing counterions and being still under the influence of considerable strong, local electrostatic fields. However the influence of this latter effect will gradually decrease with the amount of solubilized water.

It is interesting to compare these results with the w_o-dependence of particular protons of the Aerosol OT molecule. The proton in the 6th position (see Fig. 7) exhibits a strong up-field shift similar to the water proton, with decreasing solubilized amounts of water. This indicates an intense interaction of the polar part of the molecule within the interface of the micellar aggregate. The extrapolated break in the δ-w_o plot coincides reasonably well with the onset of the pronounced up-field shift which corresponds to the water proton. The difference in the bonding of D_2O and H_2O to the polar head groups of the surfactant may cause the slight variation with respect to the amount of solubilized water at constant δ. As is to be expected, the protons in the 3rd and 7th position are hardly affected by the amounts of added water. Valuable information confirming the above reported observations can moreover be gained from variations of the proton NMR

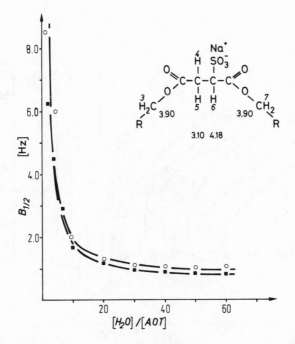

Fig. 8. Plot of half-line width ($B_{1/2}$) of the proton in the 6th
position (see insert) against the amount of solubilized water
$w_o = [H_2O]/[AOT]$, 298K.

line-widths (Fig. 8). A sharp decrease in the line-widths was observed for the water and the 6th protons in the Aerosol OT molecule.
This again offers a direct indication for the restricted mobility of
the water and the surfactant molecules with small amounts of water
(see also results from Kerr-effect measurements[13]). The apolar tails
on the contrary are almost unaffected. The mobilities of the different parts of the surfactant molecule which are due to the hydration
interactions are thus unequal and may be conveniently described by
different relaxation times (τ_c). The latter quantity may be easily
calculated from the line-widths using the expression for the spin-spin
relaxation time

$$(1/T_2)_{rot} = \pi\, B_{1/2} = (3\, \hbar^2 \gamma^4 /2\, b^6)\tau_c \tag{1}$$

where γ is the gyromagnetic ratio, $\hbar$ Planck's constant divided by
2π, $B_{1/2}$ is the half-line-width and b the inter-proton distance. Considering τ_c of the 6th proton which is located close to the interface,
the nearest neighbouring proton is either the 4th and/or the 5th
(vicinal) proton with an approximate distance of about .154 nm. If

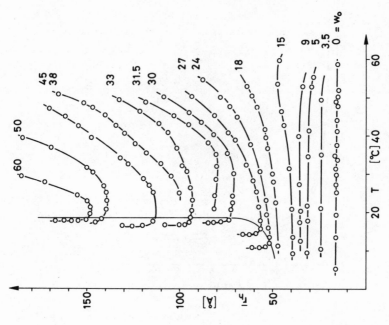

Fig. 10. Plot of the hydrodynamic radii ($\bar{r}_h$) of AOT micelles and micellar aggregates (containing solubilized water) in H_2O/ Aerosol OT/i-C_8H_8 against temperature. Parameter: $w_o = [H_2O]/[AOT]$ (15)

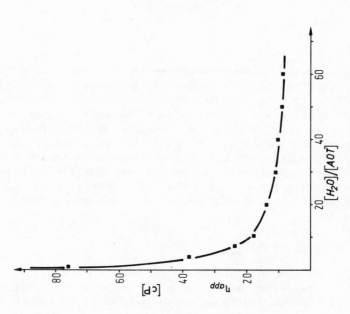

Fig. 9. Plot of apparent viscosity (η_{app}) against the amount of solubilized water $w_o = [H_2O]/(AOT]$, 298K.

Stokes-Einstein's law is applied, i.e. $\tau_c = 4\pi \eta r^3/3kT$, and assumed
that the above defined correlation time is a measure of the time required for a water molecule to rotate through an angle of one radian,
an apparent viscosity of the water core within the micellar aggregate
can be calculated as shown in Fig. 9.

At this stage of the discussion, it is worthwhile to recapitulate
the results obtained with respect to the transition from inverted
micelles to larger "closed" aggregates. A remarkable fact is the very
satisfactory coincidence regarding the w_o-values which correspond to
the breaks in the plots of Figs. 6 and 7. The same result has been
recently obtained by MARTINEK et al[14] in solubilizing 2,4-Dinitro-
phenol as acid-base indicator in Aerosol OT aggregates dissolved in
octane. The following Fig. 10 will present additional evidence for
these observations.

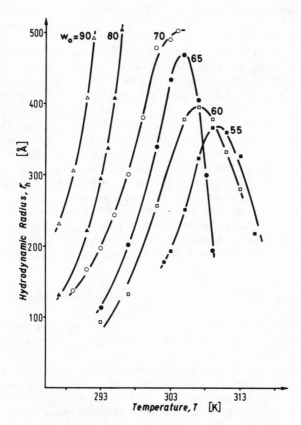

Fig. 11. Plot of the average hydrodynamic radii ($\overline{r}_h$) of micellar
aggregates (containing solubilized water) against temperature. Parameters: $w_o = [H_2O]/[AOT]$. $\overline{r}_h$-values derived from Kerr effect
measurements.

If all the information is summarized which concerns this particular w_o-range, a rather well-defined, reproducible, and unsteady transi
tion from the gel-like micellar structure to an aggregate with macroscopically describable interfacial properties can be observed. A
particularly interesting experimental survey is shown in Fig. 11. It
represents photon-correlation-spectroscopic measurements at the water/
Aerosol OT/isoctane system over the whole region from the micelles to
the microemulsion aggregates. Hydrodynamic radii versus the temperature are plotted and it is apparent at once from an inspection of the
curves that the above discussed transition has to be located at about
w_o = 10. The diagram yields additional background information regarding the phenomenological picture of the microemulsion domain presented
in Fig. 1. At low temperatures the onset of a phase transition is
evident at w_o - values above about 20. These vertical branches of the
curves corresponding to different w_o-values are the geometrical locus
of the so-called cloud-point curve (= the lower phase boundary of the
transparent region). The maxima at higher temperatures starting in
this example with w_o = 15 could not be detected due to intense scattering. If D_2O is solubilized instead of water, this higher temperature region can easily be investigated[8]. These maximum hydrodynamic
radii in microemulsions containing water can, however, be nicely
detected with Kerr-effect measurements (Fig. 11). These maxima could
be interpreted as surfactant transitions from "closed" to "open"
aggregates, i.e. lamellar, liquid crystalline phases. The latter
might represent (within the microemulsion domain) the first indication
of the phase inversion process. The maxima can also be connected by
a curve, representing the upper phase boundary of the micro-emulsion
domain. Plotted as a double logarithmic diagram a straight line
results, from which, according to the thermodynamical model, the transition entropies of the above mentioned process can be calculated.
Another hint concerning the phase transition concept is suggested by
Fig. 12, where both the electrical conductivity and the hydrodynamic
radius $(\bar{r}_h)$, versus the temperature are plotted. The nice coincidence
between the onset of the conductivity and the $\bar{r}_h$-maximum is noteworthy.

The discovery of an optical matching phenomenon (Fig. 13) in
water-in-oil microemulsions (H_2O/AOT/i-C_8H_8)[15] offered the opportu-
nity to learn more about the equilibrium properties of the surfactant
monolayers. This can be considered to be rather exceptional and is
possible due to the condition $n_{AOT} > n_{i-C_8} > n_{H_2O}$. The scattering
data could very satisfactorily be interpreted by a theoretical
model[16], considering the fact that at the matching condition the
residual scattering is solely due to fluctuations of surfactant molecules in the "equilibrium" monolayer. It was concluded from this finding that physical properties of the surfactant monolayers should be
accessible from these experiments. Hence the isothermal compressibility has been determined from the temperature dependent shift of the
optical matching condition[17]. As was to be expected, the compressibility data of the anionic surfactant (Aerosol OT) are found to range

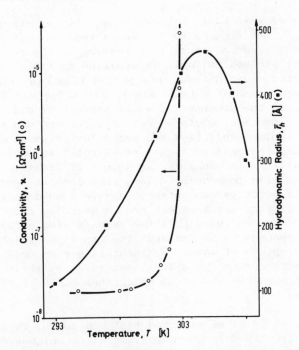

Fig. 12. Dependence of the specific electric conductivity ($\varkappa$) and average hydrodynamic radius ($\overline{r}_h$) at $w_o = [H_2O]/[AOT] = 65$ on temperature. System: H_2O/Aerosol OT/i-C_8H_8.

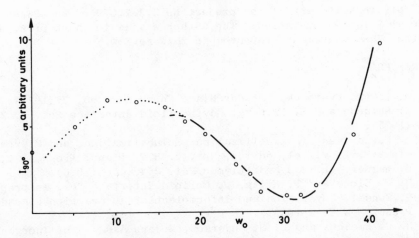

Fig. 13. Plot of the scattered intensity at right angles to the incident beam (I_{90}) against amount of solubilized water $w_o = [H_2O/[AOT]$ in H_2O/Aerosol OT/i-C_8H_8, 298K; open circles experimental points, solid line calculated according to theoretical model[16].

between those of pure hydrocarbons and aqueous electrolyte solutions. Also investigations concerning the so-called co-surfactant effect[18, 19,20] with additives atypical with respect to the conventionally used cosurfactants, yielded valuable information on the structural details of the surfactant monolayers. It appeared from the determination of t solubilization capacity and the electronic polarizability of the solu bilized water in the presence of small amounts of different organic additives like benzene, cyclohexane, nitrobenzene and carbon tetrachloride that polarizabilities and molecular volumes of the additives are determining the maximum amount of solubilized water. The higher the polarizability, the smaller the amount of additive to reach the maximum. Also with increasing molecular volume at constant polarizability, higher additive concentrations were needed to reach the solubilization capacity. From recent proton magnetic resonance experiments it could be concluded that the primary step after adding the quaternary component is to "expand" the monolayer which apparently increases the uptake of water, while at larger amounts the additives start to interfere with the solubilized water by their proper solvation interactions with the polar headgroups of the surfactant molecules.

Finally, it is to be expected that due to the rapid development of new theoretical models and experimental techniques our understanding of the microemulsion phenomenon together with many related problems within the mesophase area will improve. This will certainly apply also to the introductory remarks, since new experimental results are the best guiding-principle regarding true or semantic problems.

ACKNOWLEDGEMENT

This work is part of the project No 2.227.079 of the Swiss National Science Foundation. The author wishes to thank Dr A. Maitra for the NMR-measurements reported in this review.

REFERENCES

1. J. Th. G. Overbeek, Faraday Disc. Chem. Soc. 65, 7 (1978).
2. K. Shinoda and S. Friberg, Adv. Colloid Interface Sci. 4, 281 (1975).
3. L. E. Scriven, in Micellization, Solubilization, and Microemulsion (K. L. Mittal, edit.), Vol. 2, 877, Plenum Press, N.Y. 1977.
4. C. Wagner, Colloid and Polymer Sci. 254, 400 (1976).
5. H. F. Eicke and P. Kvita, J. Colloid Interface Sci. in prep.
6. G. Zundel, "Hydration and Intermolecular Interaction", Academic Press, New York 1969.
7. H. J. Emeléus and J. S. Anderson, Modern Aspects of Inorganic Chemistry, Rutledge and Kegan Paul Ltd., London, 386, (1960).
8. H. F. Eicke, J. Solution Chem. (1980/81) in press.
9. A. B. F. Duncan and J. A. Pople, Trans. Faraday, Soc. 49, 217, (1953).

10. H. F. Eicke, and H. Christen, Helv. Chim. Acta 61, 2258 (1978).
11. H. F. Eicke, and J. Rehak, Helv. Chim. Acta 59, 2883 (1976).
12. S. M. F. Tavernier, C. Vonk and R. Gijbels, J. Colloid Interface
     Sci. to appear (1980).
13. H. F. Eicke, and Z. Markovic, J. Colloid Interface Sci. 79, 151
     (1981); Z. Markovic, Thesis, Univ. Basel 1980.
14. A. V. Levashov, V. I. Pantin and K. Martinek, Koll. Zh. (russ.)
     No. 3, 453 (1979).
15. M. Zulauf, and H. F. Eicke, J. Phys. Chem. 83 480 (1979).
16. H. F. Eicke, and R. Kubik, Ber. Bunsenges. Phys. Chem. 84,
     37 (1980).
17. H. F. Eicke, and K. St. Nitsche, Lett. to Edit., J. Colloid
     Interf. Sci., in preparation.
18. H. F. Eicke, J. Colloid Interface Sci. 68, 440 (1979).
19. H. F. Eicke, Helv. Chim. Acta 62, 448 (1979).
20. D. Dünnenberger, unpublished results.
21. H. F. Eicke, and H. Christen, Helv. Chim. Acta 61, 2258 (1978).

Prof F. Franks: I am intrigued by your result that the Cs^+AOT stabilised system has a hydrodynamic radius r_h which is temperature dependent and seems to approach the temperature independent value (~2 nm) observed for NH_4^+ or K^+AOT stabilised systems. This cannot be accounted for in terms of double layer electrostatics but is presumably due to ion solvation effects. Have you any explanation for these observations?

Prof H. F. Eicke: It is true that the observed temperature dependence of Cs-, Rb-, and NH_4 di-2-ethylhexyl sulfosuccinates and their approach to an apparently temperature independent r_h-value is interpreted by hydration interactions between the counterions and water molecules according to the model shown in Fig. 4. The quasi-elastic light-scattering experiments show that the polydispersity of the particular salt is the greater the weaker the hydration interaction with its counterion. The reason is very probably the tendency to form non-stoichiometric aggregates due to dipole-dipole interactions (as is known from cationic surfactants with weak hydrophilic head groups). The polydispersity decreases with increasing temperature whereby the increased solubility of the surfactant monomer competes with the network building hydration interaction between counterion and sulfonate groups.

Prof B. Lindman: In your interpretation of the quasi-elastic light scattering data you use the Stokes-Einstein equation neglecting interaggregate interactions. For a low dielectric medium even a small net charge on the aggregates might give important electrostatic repulsions - would you like to comment on this point?

Prof H. F. Eicke: The specific electric conductivity of the system at a particular $w_o = 65$ (Fig. 12) is of the order of $10^{-6} \Omega^{-1} m^{-1}$.

If the hydrodynamic particle radius is assumed to be 20 nm the mobility of this particle is of the order of 2.5×10^{-7} m^2/Vs. From these figures one obtains a degree of dissociation of approximately $7 \cdot 10^{-5}$. This value is small, hence the possible effect of electrostatic repulsion is probably negligible compared to steric interactions of the aggregates. However, no such effect could be detected from the auto-correlation function. The latter was at all concentrations and solubilized amounts of water always a single exponential. It is concluded, therefore, that the Stokes-Einstein equation is still valid in the investigated concentration region. Also comparisons of the hydrodynamic radii at equal w_o-values in different concentrated surfactant solutions showed reasonable coincidence.

Dr J. F. Holzwarth: How does the change from H_2O to D_2O influence the interaction inside your aggregates?

Dr P. R. Rowland: You state a difference in the effect of D_2O and H_2O due to different hydrogen bonding energies. I find this difficult to believe. Hydrogen bonding is an electrostatic effect. The difference in energies between a proton or a deuteron bonded to oxygen in water is due to differences in vibrational zero point energies which is not the same thing. What independent evidence is there for the assertion that the charge on a proton (and hence its electrostatic effects) is different from that on a deuteron? This would be a remarkable discovery. If differences exist their interpretation should be sought in rotational and vibrational energy levels which could affect ionisation energies.

Prof H. F. Eicke: Solubilizing D_2O instead of H_2O decreases the stability of micellar aggregates in agreement with the fact that the heats of solvation of ions in D_2O are smaller than in H_2O. Consequently, the binding of a deuterium oxide molecule to the counterion of the anionic surfactant (see model, Fig. 4) is expected to be weaker, hence reducing the tendency of the surfactants to form aggregates. According to spectroscopical results and model calculations (see e.g. "The Hydrogen Bond, Recent Developments in Theory and Experiment", P. Schuster, G. Zundel, and C. Sandorfy eds., North Holland Publ. Co., Chapter 15, 1976) an additional effect of the electrostatic field of the counterion on the proton or deuteron is to be expected which should increase the symmetry of the O - H(D)...O bridge and hence its stability. This effect should be smaller in the case of a deuteron bridge.

DYNAMIC LIGHT SCATTERING FROM WATER MICROEMULSIONS IN ORGANIC

MEDIA

J. D. Nicholson, J. V. Doherty and J. H. R. Clarke

Department of Chemistry
UMIST, Manchester
P. O. Box 88, M60 1QD

INTRODUCTION

Microemulsions are thermodynamically stable apparently homogeneous dispersions of water in oil (W/O) or oil in water (O/W). These
isotropic, solubilised systems can form in the presence of surfactants,
sometimes also requiring the presence of a co-surfactant.

It is generally assumed[1] that the W/O suspended droplets are
spherical in shape with a structure approximately that shown in Fig. 1.
In many ways they are simpler systems than O/W emulsions since the
anionic "head groups" and counter ions are considered to reside at or
inside the interface of the surfactant "coat" with the aqueous core.
These droplets are therefore essentially electrically neutral and
should exhibit no long range coulombic interactions unlike their O/W
counter parts in which the counter ions disperse into the aqueous
bulk phase leading to strong electrical interactions.

Aerosol-O.T (sodium bis-2-ethyl hexyl sulphosuccinate) or AOT
(Fig. 1) is an anionic double chain surfactant capable of solubilizing
large amounts of water in organic solvents to form micro-emulsions
without the use of a co-surfactant. In this study we have used AOT to
stabilise water microemulsions in several organic solvents. AOT was
used in preference to more complicated systems such as sodium dodecyl
sulphate (SDS) and pentan-1-ol, since the alcohol in a four component
system is present in the bulk phase, surfactant layer and water core
of the microemulsion droplets simultaneously.

The technique we have used to investigate these microemulsions/
inverse micelles is Dynamic Light Scattering (DLS) which provides
direct information on the translational motion of droplets from their

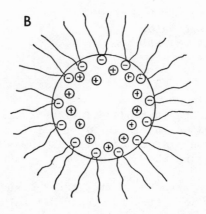

Fig. 1.   (a)   Structure of aerosol-OT.
          (b)   Model structure for water-in-oil microemulsion droplet.

mutual diffusion coefficients$^{(2,3)}$. Micellar or droplet sizes may
then be deduced from the Stokes-Einstein relation.

    The aims of the study upon which we have embarked are threefold.
Firstly we wish to characterise the sizes of microemulsion particles
and any dependencies on the mole ratio, R, of water to surfactant and
the nature of the solvent.   Secondly, it is of interest to investigate
the nature of any particle interactions in these systems, both direct
and indirect (hydrodynamic), from the dependence of diffusion coefficient on concentration.   These interactions may take many forms, from
simple hard sphere repulsive forces to rather specific attractive
effects.   The latter could arise, for example, from the entanglement
of surfactant chains on different particles.   This effect might lead

to "sticky" particle collisions or particle associations. Studies of
the concentration dependence of diffusion coefficients is also of
practical importance. These microemulsions are rather weak scatterers
(at least by comparison with many polymer suspensions) and the tendency has been to study them in rather large concentrations (volume
fractions of 5% or more have been used[4,5,6]. Under these conditions
mean particle separations are of the same order as particle diameters
and we cannot expect the simple Stokes-Einstein model for deducing
particle sizes to be reliable. The third objective concerns the
possible characterisation of polydispersity in these microemulsions.

THEORY

Analysis of fluctuations in the intensity, I, of light scattering
yields the normalised intensity auto-correlation function $g^{(2)}(t)$

$$g^{(2)}(t) = \left\langle I(o)I(t) \right\rangle \left\langle I \right\rangle^{-2} \qquad \ldots (1)$$

where the angle brackets indicate a time average. Since in our
studies the number of scattering particles is very large, Gaussian
field statistics will apply to the scattered light and the following
relation holds[2]

$$g^{(2)}(t) = 1 + C \left| g^{(1)}(t) \right|^2 \qquad \ldots (2)$$

where C is a constant close to unity depending on the experimental
conditions and $g^{(1)}(t)$ is the normalised scattered electric field
correlation function

$$g^{(1)}(t) = \left\langle E(o)E^*(t) \right\rangle \left\langle I \right\rangle^{-1} \qquad \ldots (3)$$

It is $g^{(1)}(t)$ which is the property of primary interest since it is
directly related to the motions of the scattering particles. The
total amplitude at the detector of the electric field of light single-
scattered through an angle θ by N particles can be written

$$E(K,t) \propto \sum_{i=1}^{N} A_i \exp (i\vec{K}.\vec{r}_i) \qquad \ldots (4)$$

where $\vec{K}$ is the scattering wave vector ($|\vec{K}| = \frac{4n\pi}{\lambda_o} \sin^2 \frac{\theta}{2}$), n is the
refractive index of the medium, λ_o is the wavelength in vacuuo and
$\vec{r}_i$ is the position of particle i at time t. A is the particle polari-
sability and gives the amplitude of scattering from the ith particle.

In the simple case where all the scattering particles are identical by substitution of (4) in (3) one obtains

$$g^{(1)}(t) = F(\vec{K},t)[S(\vec{K})]^{-1} \qquad \ldots (5)$$

where $F(K,t)$ is the intermediate scattering function

$$F(K,t) = \left\langle \sum_{i,j} \exp i\vec{K}.[\vec{r}_j(o) - \vec{r}_i(t)] \right\rangle \qquad \ldots (6)$$

and $S(\vec{K}) = F(\vec{K},0)$ is the structure factor. Some simplification is possible for W/O microemulsion particles. As previously mentioned these particles are expected to be uncharged and any interactions between them will be short ranged e.g. within one particle diameter. Since the particle radii are ~3 nm it is normally assumed that there will be no direct correlations in the motions of different particles beyond r_{ij} ~10 nm. These correlations will make only a small contribution to the sum of exponential terms in equation (6) since K^{-1} is of order 50 nm. All other terms for which $i \neq j$ in equation (6) will vanish in the averaging. Even though the microemulsions that are being discussed are in fact quite concentrated, to a first approximation it is justified to neglect all terms with $i \neq j$. Equation (6) then simplifies to an autocorrelation function and

$$g^{(1)}(t) = \exp i\vec{K}. \Delta \vec{r}_i(t) \qquad \ldots (7)$$

where Δr_i is the displacement of particle i in time t. Furthermore, for Brownian motion characterised by a mutual diffusion coefficient D (2,7,8).

$$g^{(1)}(t) = \exp (-DK^2 t) \qquad \ldots (8)$$

In sufficiently dilute solution $D(=D_0)$ will be identical to tracer diffusion coefficient, D_t, and according to the Stokes-Einstein model

$$D_t = kTf^{-1} \qquad \ldots (9)$$

where f is the friction coefficient and for spheres

$$f = 6\pi r_h \eta \qquad \ldots (10)$$

where η is the viscosity of the medium through which the particle diffuses and r_h is the hydrodynamic radius.

It is worth reflecting somewhat on some of the assumptions of the foregoing treatment. For water-oil microemulsions there is, in fact, substantial scattering from the solvent molecules. Although we expect solvent relaxation processes to be much faster and hence uncoupled from particle motions they do produce background scattering which statistically degrades the quality of the correlation functions. Secondly it cannot be expected that the microemulsions will be truly monodisperse so that $g^{(1)}(t)$ will be an A^2 weighted average of exponentials.

$$g^{(1)}(t) = \Sigma\, G_a \exp{-D_a \mathbf{K}^2 t} \qquad \dots (11)$$

where G_a is the normalised intensity contribution from species a.
If there is substantial polydispersity the large particles may well
dominate in $g^{(1)}(t)$. Lastly there is the question as to how dilute
the suspensions must be for equations (7), (9) and (10) to hold. This
can only be answered by studying D as a function of volume fraction
(see section 5(ii)).

EXPERIMENTAL

The technique of photon correlation spectroscopy which has rapidly developed since the advent of the laser[8,9,10] has been used
extensively to study micellar and microemulsion systems in aqueous
solutions[11,12]. The first reports of studies of water/AOT/organic
solvent systems were in 1979 by Day et al[4] and by Zulauf and
Eicke (5). In both reports data were interpreted in terms of the
second-order of intensity correlation function. The results were
obtained using the clipped correlation technique[2] in both cases. In
this article we present results obtained using both a clipped correlator (Malvern K7023 24 channel clipped correlator) and a multibit
correlator (Malvern K7025, 64 channels). The multibit correlator has
a 64 channel delay immediately preceeding the last eight channels so
that the statistical mean of the last eight correlation channels may
be taken as an experimentally determined background see equation (2).
This eliminates the arbitrariness of free-fitting the background[4,5]

The laser used in these experiments was a Spectra Physics Model
165 argon ion operating at 488 nm. The samples of the microemulsions
were contained in 1 cm^2 cross-section glass cells which, after centrifugation to remove suspended microscopic impurities (eg. dust),
were placed in a thermostatted aluminium scattering cell holder with
temperature control to $\pm$ 0.5°C. The photomultiplier used to detect
the scattered light was an ITT FW 130. Correlation functions could
be measured over a range of angles from 10° to 40° and from 50° to
130° through the front and side faces of the scattering cell respectively.

The use of a refractive-index matching liquid was deliberately
avoided, instead corrections based on Snell's Law of Refraction were
made to obtain the true angle of scattering for all angles other than
at 90°(4).

The K7025 correlator was interfaced to an RML 380Z 48K micro-
computer for processing. Data was stored on mini-floppy disc.

The microemulsions were prepared by dissolving a weighed quantity
of dried AOT (Fluka, Switzerland) in analytical reagent grade organic
solvent (BDH, England).

A weighed quality of triply distilled water was then syringed
into the AOT solutions. Solubilization by shaking the solution
resulted in a transparent solution. Various solutions of constant
water/surfactant molar ratio, R, were prepared by careful dilution of
the stock solution with organic solvent. The volume fractions, ϕ,
of micelles reported here were obtained by subtracting the added
solvent volume from that of the solution. This assumes that all
the water is solubilized in the microemulsion droplets and the amount
of AOT present as surfactant monomers is negligible in comparison
with the aggregated surfactant. This is reasonable since the CMC of
AOT in the organic solvents used is much smaller than the AOT concentrations used in this study. Typically the CMC lies between 10^{-3} and
10^{-4} mol dm^{-3}.

DATA ANALYSIS

The results presented in section 5(i) were analysed in terms of
the second order or intensity correlation function, $g^{(2)}(t)$. The
natural logarithm of the correlation function minus the background
signal was fitted to a straight line using the method of least squares
with the dc level as a free parameter. Since the introduction of the
multibit correlator and the direct method of background estimation,
data have been analysed in terms of the normalised electric field
correlation function, $g^{(1)}(t)$, obtained from $g^{(2)}(t)$ through the
Siegert relation, equation (2).

Several methods of analysing $g^{(1)}(t)$ have been used. Firstly
data were fitted to a single exponential using a weighted linear
least squares procedure for $\ln g(t)$. Since $g(1)(t)$ or $g(2)(t)$ are
obtained after subtracting a constant signal the relative statistical
error will vary from the initial to the final points. Each point
should be weighted, therefore, by the inverse of its variance[13,14].
Assuming the same statistical uncertainty for each point on a particular measured correlation function then a normalised weighting factor
(W_i) can be defined for the i'th point so that

$$W_i = (y_i - b)^2 / N^{-1} \sum_{i}^{N} (y_i - b)^2 \qquad \ldots(12)$$

where y_i is the store contents of the ith correlation channel (total
number N) and b is the background.

It was found generally that $g^{(1)}(t)$ was significantly non-
exponential and that the deviation varied in a systematic manner.
One possible reason for this is the existence of polydispersity
giving rise to a sum of exponentials in $g(1)(t)$, see equation (11).
Under these conditions $g^{(1)}(t)$ can be analysed using the method of
cumulants[15,2].

$$\ln g^{(1)}(t) = -\overline{\Gamma} t + 1/2 \left(\frac{\mu_2}{\overline{\Gamma}^2}\right) (\overline{\Gamma} t)^2 - \qquad \ldots(13)$$

where $\overline{\Gamma}$ is the mean inverse relaxation time ($=\overline{D}K^2$) and the μ's are moments of the normalised distribution about the mean. Equation (13) is exact when all terms are retained. In practice only the first two terms can be given statistical significance for DLS data, so the analysis is only useful for narrow distributions ($\mu_2/\overline{\Gamma}^2 < 0.25$). Only if the quadratic term is zero to within experimental error ($\mu_2/\overline{\Gamma}^2 \simeq 0.01$) can data be said to be exponential. The variance $\mu_2/\overline{\Gamma}^2$ is often called[16] the "index of polydispersity". However, non-exponentiality can arise for other reasons in strongly interacting solutions[17]. Experimental data were fitted for 48 points to a quadratic in t according to equation (13), using the weighted least-squares procedure. In most cases values of $\mu_2/\overline{\Gamma}^2$ were between 0.1 and 0.25 so that we feel justified in terminating the series (13) after the 2nd term.

For some of the most concentrated microemulsions it was found that the quadratic fit was rather poor and values of $\mu_2/\overline{\Gamma}^2$ were quite large (0.3 or more) and an alternative fitting procedure was adopted. In the case of the $g^{(1)}(t)$ reported in Fig. (4b) for $\emptyset = 0.38$, R = 30, for instance, the correlation function was divided into two regions. The last 20 points of $\log_e g^{(1)}(t)$ (the tail) were fitted to a straight line and the exponential it represented was subtracted from the experimental data. The residuals were fitted to an exponential over the first 10 points. This technique requires that the short time exponential has essentially decayed to zero before commencing the tail fit so an iterative procedure is necessary for self-consistency. The method can only be meaningful for well-separated exponentials.

It may be worth mentioning that Chu et al[18,19] have developed an alternative histogram method of data analysis for PCS which they claim to be perfectly general but has the advantage over the cumulant method of being able to distinguish between bimodal distributions. We have not attempted this method of analysis.

RESULTS AND DISCUSSION

Particle Sizes and Solvent Effects

Microemulsions with varying water content but with constant surfactant concentration were studied in various solvents. Hydrodynamic radii were calculated from the observed diffusion coefficients assuming the validity of the Stokes-Einstein relation (equations (9) and (10). These data were obtained using the 24-channel single-clipped correlator, fitting the correlation functions to a single exponential plus a constant background (see section (4)). The results, shown in Fig. 2 are directly comparable with previous data in other solvents[4,5]. The precision of diffusion coefficients is $\pm$ ~5% for the current data.

The salient trends in Fig. 2 are as follows:

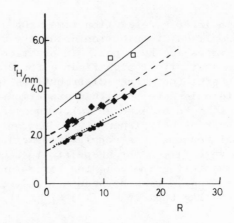

Fig. 2. Variation of apparent hydrodynamic radii, r_H with water to
surfactant molar ratio $\underline{R}$ for solutions 0.1 mol dm^{-3} in AOT, as
determined by dynamic light scattering at 20°C $\pm 1^{\circ}$C.
   ● - toluene as solvent
   ◆ - n-heptane as solvent
   □ - cyclohexane as solvent
broken line, iso-octane as solvent[5]
dotted line, n-heptane as solvent, ultracentrifuge data (4).

1. For all solvents the effective hydrodynamic radii of the micelles/
microemulsion droplets increase with increasing water-to-surfactant
ratio, R. This increase is approximately linear over the R range
studied in all three cases (although no firm conclusion may be made
concerning cyclohexane as the solvent since only three molar ratios
were used (scattering from these solutions was extremely weak). If the
thickness of the surfactant layer (ℓ) remained constant as additional
water was added to the microemulsions in any particular solvent, one
may have expected $\overline{r}_H \propto R^{1/3} + \ell$ dependence according to the simple
model depicted in Fig. 1. That this is not the case suggests that
the surfactant layer decreases in thickness and expands in surface
area, as R increases, which is entirely reasonable as the same amount
of AOT must cover a greater area at large R.

2. The effective hydrodynamic radius is seen to depend on the solvent
used. For a fixed R value, $\overline{r}_H$ is greatest in cyclohexane and smallest
in toluene. A likely explanation of these results is that the microemulsion particles themselves may vary in size due to differing
amounts of solvent adsorption or actual penetration into the surfactant layer of the microemulsion particles. The situation may be clari-
fied by the use of some complementary technique to determine the size
of the water core and the thickness of the surfactant layer separately,
such as Low Angle Neutron Scattering.

Particle Interactions

In order to investigate the effect on diffusion of interactions between different particles, microemulsions of constant water/surfactant ratios were studied as a function of volume fraction in n-heptane. Low R values were chosen to maintain the systems in the 'well-behaved' region where we expect stable, water containing, reversed micelles to be formed[4,5]. In addition we shall assume that the particle sizes remain unchanged with volume fraction. Typical results are shown in Fig. 3. It is seen that as the volume fraction increases, so the diffusion coefficient decreases. The effect is substantial. From a purely empirical point of view extrapolation to $\emptyset = 0$ should be used to obtain a diffusion coefficient appropriate to the Stokes-Einstein relation (equations (9) and (10)). At $\emptyset = 0.11$, corresponding to 0.13 mol dm^{-3} surfactant solutions, the error in using the observed value of D in place of D_o is 18.5%. Quite fortuitously this is largely cancelled in the use of equation (10) by an increase of ~25% in η as compared with infinite dilution.

There is little doubt that the decrease in D and increase in η are the results of increasing particle interactions as $\emptyset$ increases. This decrease is linear at low volume fractions and can be represented by the equation

$$D = D_o \ (1 + B\emptyset) \qquad\qquad\qquad ...(14)$$

where we have found B = -1.7

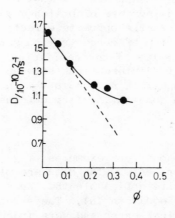

Fig. 3. Variation of mean diffusion coefficients (obtained using cumulants analysis) with volume fraction $\emptyset$ in n-heptane for a water-to-surfactant ratio of 11.2. The slope of the linear extrapolation to infinite dilution is -1.7.

Similar behaviour has been observed previously for other W/O micro-emulsions[20,21]. It must be expected that interactions will be short ranged by comparison with the particle sizes (as a first approximation one might consider them to behave as hard spheres). This is a quite different situation to that encountered in aqueous colloidal systems where as a result of a net charge on the particle outer surfaces there can be very strong and long-ranged coulombic forces.

There have been several theoretical approaches towards predicting the dependence of D on volume fraction for spherical particles in viscous media[8,22-26]. One approach[22] starts with a generalised Stokes-Einstein equation

$$D = f(c)^{-1}(d\pi/dc) \qquad \qquad \ldots(15)$$

where $d\pi/dc$ is the osmotic - compressibility ($= kT$ in the ideal dilute solution limit) which generally depends on direct particle—particle interactions. f_c is a hydrodynamic friction coefficient for mutual diffusion. Particle interactions can affect $f(c)$ indirectly since solvent fluctuations around one particle depend on the distribution and dynamics of other particles. Other approaches[24,25] have attempted a more detailed and general analysis of the interactions. Unfortunately all of the predictions apply only to very dilute solutions where interparticle separations are large compared to particle sizes. For the microemulsions discussed here and elsewhere[4-6,19-21] the volume fraction is never smaller than ~0.05 corresponding to mean separations of 3-4 particle radii. Substantial local structuring must therefore be expected and under these conditions the theoretical problem remains unsolved.

In dilute systems it appears[23] that repulsive interactions tend to cause a slight increase of D with Ø whereas the introduction of attractive forces has the opposite effect, since they will tend to slow down the dissipation of concentration gradients[24]. Our observation of a negative value of the coefficient B may be indicative of some specific attractive interactions between particles. We have speculated on their possible nature in the introduction but, as yet, it is not possible to come to any firm conclusions.

Size Fluctuations

In Fig. 4. are shown four examples of $g^{(1)}(t)$ obtained from our light scattering experiments. The data are plotted in semi-logarithmic form and it is quite noticeable that none is exactly linear as would be predicted by equation (8). The effects are quite outside the limits of statistical error and were independent of centrifuging times for any particular sample (suggesting that suspended dust particles etc. are not responsible). One possible conclusion is that we are detecting the polydispersity of the samples. Analysis through the method of cumulants (see section 4) would suggest size variances

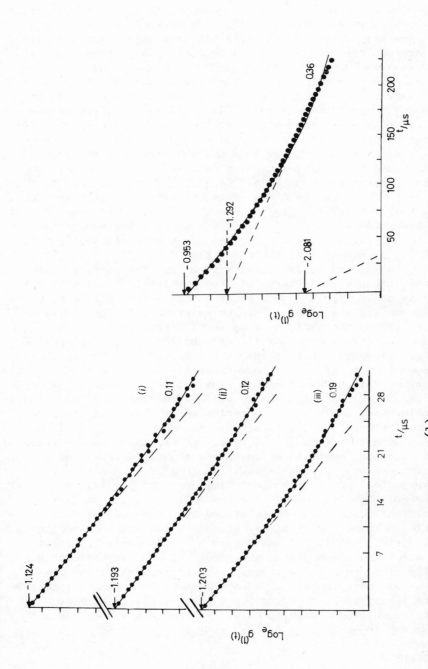

Fig. 4. Semi-logarithmic plots of $g^{(1)}(t)$ against t for selected w/o microemulsions. $\emptyset$ is volume fraction, R is water to surfactant ratio. (a) (i) R = 11, $\emptyset$ = 0.11 (b) R = 30, $\emptyset$ = 0.38 (ii) R = 11, $\emptyset$ = 0.22 (iii) R = 11, $\emptyset$ = 0.34 with intercepts at t=0 as indicated. Values of $\mu_2/\bar{\Gamma}^2$ are also shown. For (a), broken lines are linear fit to the first 5 points. For (b), broken lines represent the components of a two exponential fit (see section 4).

Solid lines are fit to equation (13), with intercepts at t=0 as indicated.

of 8-20% for the R = 11.2 suspensions if we assume normal distributions (the typical error in $\bar{\Gamma}$, (see equation (13)), due to uncertainty in the background was less than 1%). It is worth noting here
that the Z-averaged diffusion coefficients so obtained are 13% different on average from those obtained by forcing an exponential fit
with the background as a free parameter in the correlation
functions (see section 4). For the low R value systems there is only
a small difference between a dilute and concentrated suspension as
far as the deviation from exponential in $g^{(1)}(t)$. Particle interactions seem to have no great effect on the distribution of particle
sizes. Eventually, however, at very high volume fractions (approach-
ing the inversion point) and for high R values the $g^{(1)}(t)$ become
highly non-exponential in form and any explanation in terms of simple
polydispersity seems inappropriate. It is, in fact, possible to
parametrise the functions as a sum of two exponentials (see section 4)
which differ in relaxation time by a factor of ~5. Functions of this
type have been observed[16,17,27,28] for aqueous latex suspensions
with strong electrical repulsive forces and inter-particle separations
of order K^{-1}. In these cases the short time decay of $g^{(1)}(t)$ [for t
less than τ_I, the characteristic relaxation time for particle inter-
actions] was interpreted in terms of free particle diffusion whilst
the long time decay [for K^{-1} much greater than interparticle spacings]
is due to cooperative motions. For the water-in-oil microemulsions
we expect particle interactions to be short ranged so that t >> τ_I
even for the short time decay of $g^{(1)}(t)$ and the simple explanation
for the short time behaviour is inappropriate. More probably the
cause is some form of effective polydispersity resulting from particle
associations or "sticky" collisions. The collision rate, τ_c^{-1}, of
particles is extremely high at large volume fractions (and this could
lead to coalescence of two or more particles at a time if the duration of a collision, τ_{stick}, is of the same order as τ_c. Since
τ_c is very much less than $g^{(1)}(t)$ decay rates, this would correspond
to a "fast exchange limit" in which only the average result of a
range of complex interactions is manifest in $g^{(1)}(t)$. Recently it
has been suggested[29] that the long time decay of $g^{(1)}(t)$ in strongly
interacting colloidal systems in the low K limit is due to distinct
polydispersity fluctuations characterised by a "tracer" diffusion
coefficient and uncoupled from the collective fluctuations responsible
for mutual diffusion[23]. It was argued[29] that particles might
differ in size (and hence scattering power) without significantly
changing the (long range) electrical interactions due to surface
charge. For W/O microemulsions, however, the (short range) interactions are likely to be a strong function of particle size so that
any distinction between polydispersity fluctuations and collective
effects is hard to envisage.

ACKNOWLEDGEMENTS

    The authors are grateful to Mr C. Ward for supplying some of the
data included in Fig. 2.

The authors acknowledge financial support from Esso Chemical Research and from the Science Research Council.

REFERENCES

1. M. B. Mathews and E. Hirschhorn, J. Colloid Sci. **8**, 86 (1953).
2. P. N. Pusey and J. M. Vaughan, in "Dielectric and Related Phenomena" (Chemical Society Specialist Periodical Report, 1975) vol. II p. 48.
3. J. V. Doherty and J. H. R. Clarke, Sci. Prog. Oxf. **66**, 385, (1980).
4. R. A. Day, B. H. Robinson, J. H. R. Clarke and J. V. Doherty, J. Chem. Soc. Faraday Transactions I, **75**, 132 (1979).
5. M. Zulauf and H. F. Eicke, J. Phys. Chem., **83**, 480, (1979).
6. E. Sein, J. R. Lalanne, J. Buchert and S. Kielich, J. Coll. Interface Sci., **72**, 363 (1979).
7. A. Einstein, "Investigations on the Theory of the Brownian Movement", Dover, 1956.
8. B. J. Berne and R. Pecora, "Dynamic Light Scattering", Wiley, 1976.
9. B. Chu, "Laser Light Scattering", Academic, 1974.
10. H. Z. Cummins and E. R. Pike (eds) (a) "Photon Correlation Spectroscopy and Light Beating Spectroscopy", (b) "Photon Correlation Spectroscopy and Velocimetry" Proc. NATO ASI Plenum, (a) 1974, (b) 1977.
11. N. A. Mazer, G. B. Benedek and M. C. Carey, (a) J. Phys. Chem., **80**, 1075 (1976), (b) in "Micellization, Solubilization and Micro-emulsions", Vol. 1, ed., K. L. Mittal, Plenum, 1977.
12. M. Corti and V. Degiorgio, (a) Chem. Phys. Lett. **49**, 141, (1977); (b) Chem. Phys. Lett. **53**, 237, (1978); (c) in ref. 10(b) p. 450, (d) Annales de Physique (Paris) **3**, 303 (1978).
13. P. G. Guest "Numerical Methods of Curve Analysis" Cambridge UP, 1961.
14. O. L. Davies and P. L. Goldsmith (eds) "Statistical Methods of Research and Production", 4th Edn., Oliver and Boyd, 1972.
15. D. E. Koppel, J. Chem. Phys. **57**, 4814 (1972).
16. P. N. Pusey, J. Phys. A., **8**, 1433, (1975).
17. P. N. Pusey, Phil. Trans. Roy. Soc. Lond. A, **293**, 429 (1979).
18. (a) Z. Gulari, E. Gulari, Y. Tsunashima and B. Chu, J. Chem. Phys., **70**, 3965, (1979).
    (b) F. C. Chen, A. Yeh and B. Chu, J. Chem. Phys. **66**, 1290, (1977)
19. E. Gulari, B. Bedwell and S. Alkhafaji, J. Colloid and Interface Sci., **77**, 202, (1980).
20. A. M. Cazabat, D. Langevin and A. Pouchelon, J. Colloid and Interface Sci., **73**, 1. (1980).
21. R. Finsy, A. Devriese and H. Lekkerkerker, J. Chem. Soc., Faraday II, **76**, 767 (1980).
22. G. D. J. Phillies, J. Chem. Phys. **60**, 976, (1974); **62**, 3925 (1975), **67**, 4690 (1977).
23. G. K. Batchelor, J. Fluid Mech., **74**, 1. (1976).

24. J. L. Anderson and C. C. Reed, J. Chem. Phys., 64, 3240 (1976).
25. B. U. Felderhoff, J. Phys. A., 11, 929, (1978).
26. B. J. Ackerson, J. Chem. Phys., 69, 684, (1978).
27. J. C. Brown, P. N. Pusey, J. W. Goodwin and R. H. Ottewill,
     J. Phys. A., 8, 664 (1975).
28. P. N. Pusey, J. Phys. A., 11, 119 (1978).
29. M. B. Weissman, J. Chem. Phys., 72, 231 (1980).

DISCUSSION

Dr E. Dickinson: In addition to the effects of polydispersity and particle interactions, light scattering from concentrated systems is often complicated by multiple-scattering phenomena. Was multiple scattering a complicating factor in the analysis of your results?

Dr J. H. R. Clarke: These microemulsions scatter light only very weakly compared with most colloidal systems. The solutions are completely clear and transparent. We do not expect multiple scattering to be significant even for the most concentrated systems.

Dr I. D. Robb: Are the fluctuations in polydispersity (as noticed by Pusey) important here?

Dr J. H. R. Clarke: If polydispersity is present then there certainly will be associated fluctuations. However for W/O microemulsions it is questionable whether one can consider them as a separate relaxation mode uncoupled from the collective number fluctuations (which are always present) in the manner suggested by Weissman (and adopted by Pusey) for very dilute aqueous suspensions of latex spheres.

Dr G Gähwiller: Dynamic light scattering technique measures the translational diffusion of particles. Since micelles are continuously exchanging molecules with their surrounding will the translational motion of the micelles be perturbed by this rapid exchange? If yes, how would it affect the interpretation of your results?

Dr J. H. R. Clarke: This molecular exchange between monomer and micelle could affect the motion of the micelles. This could be described as a viscosity effect or a change in the boundary conditions for flow. I am not aware of any theory dealing with such an effect.

Prof. M. Kahlweit: What are the interfacial tensions in these systems?

Dr J. H. R. Clarke: The interfacial tensions are generally low as is to be expected (for the AOT liquid hydrocarbon chain-water interface, the interfacial tension is about 5×10^{-2} Jm^{-2}).

Prof. F. Franks: Your measurements should enable you to study rotational diffusion which is expected to show a different concentration dependence from translational diffusion. It should also provide information about the particle shape except when particles are spherical. Have you studied rotational diffusion?

Dr J. H. R. Clarke: Rotational diffusion may be detected by light scattering only for anistropically polarisable (i.e. non-spherical) particles. One would expect significant depolarised scattering from such systems. We have not observed any significant depolarised scattering from the present systems that can be ascribed to the suspended particles.

FORMATION AND STRUCTURE OF FOUR-COMPONENT SYSTEMS CONTAINING

POLYMERIC SURFACTANTS

F. Candau and F. Ballet

Centre de Recherches sur les Macromolecules, CNRS
6, rue Boussingault
67083 Strasbourg
Cedex, France

INTRODUCTION

Block and graft copolymers exhibit colloid properties very
similar to those of soaps and nonionic surfactants. For both types
of emulsifiers, the colloid behaviour arises from segregation effects
related to the incompatibility of the hydrophilic and lipophilic parts
of their molecules.

If a copolymer is dispersed in a solvent which dissolves select-
ively one sequence and is a precipitant of the other, a microphase
separation occurs between unlike copolymer sequences. In concentrated
solutions, mesomorphic phases are produced[1] while in dilute solutions micellar particles are formed. These micelles may be monomole-
cular, if the copolymer molecules are molecularly dispersed in the
solution and polymolecular if they are associated.

In the simplest situation, the micelles consist of a compact core
of the poorly soluble polymer component prevented from precipitation
by the outer shell containing the solvated sequences[2,3].

Another aspect related to the microsegregation phenomenon is the
ability of amphiphilic copolymers to solubilize water-oil mixtures in
the presence of an alcohol[4-6]. Recent studies[7] have demonstrated
some similarities between the microemulsifying properties of poly-
styrene-poly-(ethyleneoxide) (PS-PEO) graft copolymers and small nonionic surfactants. More specifically, the effect of temperature and
alcohol on the solubilization of water in non-aqueous solutions of
these polymeric emulsifiers has been investigated in detail. The
single phase domains observed in these systems may consist of either

49

anisotropic phases[8] or isotropic micellar solutions.

In this paper, we describe the different types of structures encountered for water-toluene mixtures stabilized by PS-PEO graft copolymers in the presence of 2-propanol. The main techniques used in this work were dialysis experiments, X-ray diffraction and optical microscopy.

MATERIALS AND TECHNIQUES

Materials

Monodisperse graft copolymers homogeneous in composition were prepared via anionic polymerization; they are composed of a hydrophobic polystyrene (PS) backbone and hydrophilic poly(ethyleneoxide) (PEO) grafts. The method of preparation described in a previous paper[9] allows us to obtain copolymers with different lengths of backbones as well as a variable number and length of branches. The characteristics of the two samples used in this study are listed in Table I.

Microemulsions were prepared by slow addition of the cosurfactant (2-propanol) to the water-toluene-copolymer emulsions until transparency was obtained. Samples were prepared by weight (accuracy $\pm$ 0.001g) and then mixed thoroughly on a vibromixer.

Dialysis Experiments have been performed following a procedure already described[10]. A dialysis equilibrium is established between the microemulsion and the ternary solvent mixture through a semi-permeable membrane. The measurement by gas chromatography of the weight composition of the ternary solvent mixture before and after dialysis equilibrium leads to a precise determination of the composition of the external phase surrounding the micelles.

Table 1

Structural Characteristics of Graft Copolymers

Sample	M_w (PS backbone)	M_w (PEO graft)	$\overline{P}$ (average number grafts)	M_w (copolymer)	wt% PS in COP
A4	18 200	2 100	9	38 400	49
A7	18 200	7 800	6.5	75 000	26

Table II

Compositions of the Continuous Phases for Some Quaternary Systems
Located in Areas I and II, as determined from Dialysis Experiments.

		Composition (wt%) of the quaternary system	Composition (wt%) of the solvent mixture in the system	Composition (wt%) of the continuous phase
	Syst. A			
	cop. A4	8.1		
	WATER	9.6	10.5	7.7
A	Tol.	48.1	52.3	53.7
R	2-P	34.2	37.2	38.6
E				
A	**Syst. A'**			
A	cop. A7	4.7		
I	WATER	9.4	9.9	7.1
	Tol.	46.8	49.1	53.3
	2-P	39.1	41.0	39.6
	Cop. A7	9.2		
	WATER	9.6	10.6	5.5
	Tol.	47.8	52.6	58.5
	2-P	33.5	36.9	36.0
	Syst. B			
	cop. A4	14.7		
A	WATER	12.3	14.4	0.8
R	Tol.	61.3	71.9	88.2
E	2-P	11.7	13.7	11.0
A				
	Cop. A7	12.7		
II	WATER	10.4	11.9	2.3
	Tol.	51.8	59.4	76.5
	2-P	25.1	28.7	21.2
	Cop. A7	13.4		
	WATER	11.2	12.9	2.0
	Tol.	55.8	64.4	77.4
	2-P	19.6	22.6	20.6

X-Ray Diffraction experiments (low angle) have been performed with a
Guinier Camera. The X-ray beam is monochromatized and focused by a
bent quartz crystal, which isolates the Cu-α_1 line (λ=1.54 Å). The
liquid specimens were introduced into thin wall capillary tubes, 1mm
in diameter, and the tubes were sealed in an oxygen gas flame. The
sample-to-film distance was 335mm.

The Bragg spacing was obtained by applying Bragg's law
d = n λ /2sin θ (n = 1 for first order diffraction)

Optical Microscopy. Samples of the solution were introduced into
rectangular optical capillaries of different optical pathlengths. The
capillaries were then sealed with a fast setting two component epoxy
resin. Examination of the samples was conducted on a microscope
(Leitz) between crossed polarizers. In the case of orientated mesomorphic phases, the sign and the order of magnitude of the birefringence Δn could be determined using a first-order-red gypsum plate;
accurate measurements of Δn were performed with a Berek compensator:

$$\Delta n = \frac{\Gamma}{d}$$

where Γ is the phase shift and d the thickness of the capillary.

EXPERIMENTAL RESULTS

The phase diagrams of the quaternary systems investigated here
may be represented, at constant pressure and temperature, by a tetrahedron in which each peak corresponds to one component of the system.
In order to facilitate the comprehension of these diagrams, we have
made triangular sections of the tetrahedron, keeping constant the
weight percent of copolymer with respect to the total weight of (water
+ toluene). Fig 1 and 2 show the pseudo-ternary phase diagrams
(triangles 2-P, T', W') thus obtained for samples A4 and A7 at room
temperature.

The hatched areas (IV) refer to milky emulsions. The domains I,
II, III define the region of the existence of homogeneous and thermodynamically stable systems. Phases I and II are optically isotropic
while systems III exhibit an optical birefringence and correspond to
liquid-crystalline phases. In the following, the structural characteristics of the monophasic domains located in the different regions
will be discussed separately.

Systems I

The characteristics of the transparent systems located in the
vicinity and above the mutual solubility curve of the three solvents
without copolymer (see fig 1 and 2, triangles 2P-T-W) have been
described in detail elsewhere[13]. In this domain, the composition of

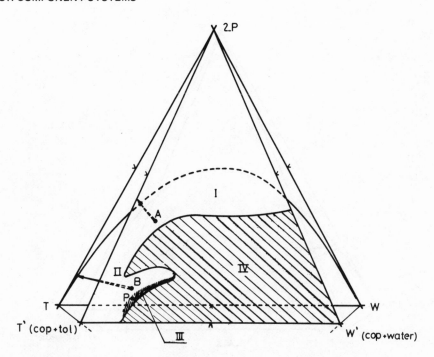

Fig. 1. Pseudo-ternary phase diagram of systems A4 at 20°C. The
wt% copolymer concentration with respect to the total weight of
(water + toluene) is Y = 0.25.
---- mutual solubility curve of the ternary solvent mixture in the
triangular plane 2-P T.W.
For sake of simplicity, the systems A and B are represented in the
same section (Y = 0.14 and 0.20 respectively, see table II).

the external phase outside the droplets as determined from dialysis
experiments, does not differ appreciably from the overall composition
of the system. This is shown in Fig. 1 and 2 where the points A and
A' refer to the overall compositions of two systems A4 and A7 respectively and the tips of the arrows to the compositions of their continuous phases respectively. In this regime, the role of the copolymer
is mainly to enhance the water-oil solubility owing to the preferential solvation of its two segregated components by the solvent mixture.
This phenomenon is similar to that already observed by several
authors[11,12] in systems involving polymers or copolymers in mixed
solvents.

The micelles may be thus depicted as a model of two concentric
spheres. One can reasonably assume that the particles consist of a

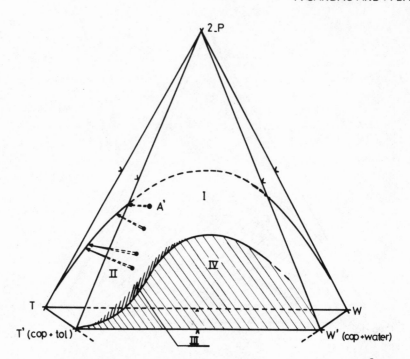

Fig. 2. Pseudo-ternary phase diagram of systems A7 at 20°C (Y=0.32)
The compositions of the four systems represented in the same triangular
section are given in table II.

hard core of polystyrene more or less collapsed covered with a layer
of poly(ethyleneoxide) which acts as a barrier to prevent contact
between polystyrene and outside water.

The sizes, the molecular weights and the aggregation numbers of
the copolymer in the dispersed particles have been determined using
small angle neutron scattering, quasi-elastic light scattering and
viscosity measurements. It was shown that in the water rich area of
the diagrams, the particles are compact with high aggregation numbers
and large dimensions (~500Å) while in the toluene rich area, the
particles are mono or bimolecular, small in size (~150Å) with a fairly
high degree of swelling. These results have been explained from considerations based on the relative compatibility between the two components of the copolymer and the solvents[13].

Systems II

The area II appears for relatively high copolymer concentrations

(>12%/system) and is mainly located in the left part of the phase
diagram (toluene-rich-area). Its formation requires much less cosurfactant, as shown in fig. 1 and 2. Information on the structure of
the particles dispersed in these systems is provided by dialysis
experiments. Let us consider for instance the systems represented by
points A and B (see fig. 1), which correspond to the same toluene/
water ratio but differ by the alcohol and copolymer contents. The
compositions of their continuous phases, given by the tips of the
arrows are reported in table II. It can be seen that for point A,
the composition of the continuous phase is close to that of the
initial microemulsion, while almost no water is present in the continuous phase of system B. This result demonstrates that water is
trapped within the copolymer droplets, implying an inverse micellar
structure, with a PEO core swollen par water, surrounded by a PS
enveloppe. Similar results are obtained for sample A7 (cf fig. 2 and
table II). However, contrary to the first example considered where
the domain IV (multiphasic) is crossed when passing from system A to
system B by increasing the alcohol content, there is not for sample
A7 a distinct boundary between regions I and II (fig. 2). The
dialysis experiments still show a significant change of the composition of the continuous phase at a given water/toluene ratio as shown
in table II (see also fig. 2.).

     Clearer evidence of a transition between these two regions is
given by considering the amount of alcohol required for the formation
of transparent systems, as a function of the copolymer concentration.
This is illustrated in fig. 3; for low copolymer concentrations, only
systems I can be formed. The coexistence of systems I and II appears
at a threshold copolymer concentration of the order of 0.11/system
for sample A4 and 0.145 for sample A7.

     It can be remarked that contrary to systems I, systems II exhibit
the same general features (structure and composition) as classical
water in oil microemulsions formed from soaps or nonionic surfactants[14].

Systems III

     The characteristics and the domain of the existence of the aniso-
tropic systems III are strongly dependent on the chemical composition
of the copolymer and on the temperature.

Sample A7: The area describing the mesomorphic phases formed from
sample A7 extends close to the phase separation as shown in fig. 2.
This behaviour has already been observed for other surfactant systems
in continuous oil phases[15,16]. In the polarizing microscope,
samples have been found to exhibit textures reminiscent of those frequently observed with classical liquid crystals. One example of a
specific texture is shown in fig. 4. The corresponding X-ray pattern
contains 2 diffraction bands in which the bands are related by a $\sqrt{3}$

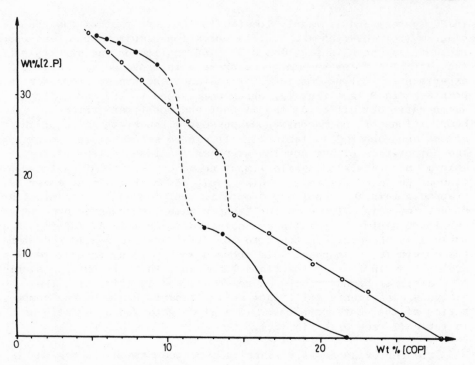

Fig. 3. Percentage of 2-propanol required for the formation of monophasic systems as a function of the copolymer concentration
● systems A4   o systems A7

factor, denoting an hexagonal array of indefinite cylinders. It can
be assumed that the PEO chains fill with water the interior of the
cylinders and the PS sequences lie on the surface separating the two
immiscible solvents. As for 2-propanol, it should be distributed
between both phases owing to its partition coefficient.

     The Bragg spacings d, i.e. the distance between the axes of the
cylinders do not vary much with the copolymer concentration and the
location of the system in the phase diagram. Their values range from
300 to 400 Å. We have reported in table III, as an example, the
values of d obtained for some systems at different copolymer concentrations. These systems are located right above the transition line
between the cream emulsion and the monophasic domain and have been
obtained after titration with 2-propanol of the toluene-water-copoly-
mer emulsions. The random distribution of the d values presumably
results from the experimental difficulty to realize an accurate titration of the microemulsions. Although it was not possible to establish

in a quantitative way the variation of d with the alcohol content, we
observed qualitatively that the Bragg spacing decreases with the
alcohol content, indicating a shrinking of the copolymer. For higher
alcohol amounts, only one band is observed denoting possibly that the
cylinders have turned into uniform spheres.

It should also be noticed that the Bragg spacing values are
larger than those generally measured for classical systems formed with
soaps [17,18] but are compatible with the data found in literature
concerning block copolymers in solution of a selective solvent for one
sequence [1].

As the systems III are relatively fluid, they can be orientated
by forcing them to flow into rectangular optical capillaries, under
an excess pressure of nitrogen between 0 and 10cm Hg, depending on the
viscosity of the samples. Observations on the optical microscope provided us information on the uniformity of their orientation and on
their direction with respect to that of the flow. The liquid-crystalline samples generally show a rapid reorientation on flowing in capillaries. They behave like a liquid-crystalline plate, with the orientation of the optical axis parallel to the direction of the flow. The
sign of the birefringence is always positive. It is of interest that
these orientated systems keep their 45° birefringence for hours; the
value of the phase shift remains constant, even after stopping the
flow.

The values of the birefringence Δn, measured with a Berek compensator are given in table III. It can be seen that as for the Bragg
spacing, Δn does not show any regular variation with the polymer concentration and is of the order of $2.5.10^{-4}$. These observations confirm the X-ray results, i.e. the existence of cylinders which are
orientated in a direction parallel to that of the flow, as already
found for nonionic systems [18].

Sample A4: These systems are also located in a small region close to
the transition line. When moving away from this region by addition
for instance of alcohol, the solutions become optically isotropic, as
shown by microscopic examination between crossed polarizers. Intermediate areas of coexisting isotropic and anisotropic phases may eventually be observed.

In view of our present results concerning systems A4, only mesomorphic phases characteristic of a lamellar structure have been
obtained. This structure consists of parallel and equidistant sheets.
Each sheet results from the superposition of two layers. One layer
contains the PS backbones swollen by toluene while the other contains
the PEO grafts in water, the alcohol existing presumably in both
phases. The X-ray patterns contain 2 diffraction lines the reciprocal
Bragg spacings of which are in the ratio 1:2. For a system corresponding to point P in fig. 1, the Bragg spacing d is equal to 280 Å.

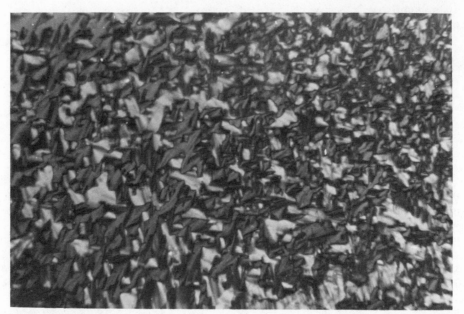

Fig. 4. Example of a texture observed for a cylindrical structure
(system A7) between crossed polarizers (G=260).

Table III

Values of the birefringence and the Bragg spacings for systems A7
at different copolymer concentrations (ponderal ratio tolulene/water =

wt % cop. A7 (/ Syst.)	wt % 2-P (/ Syst.)	d (Å) (Bragg spacing)	Δn 10^4
14.3	18.3	370 (1 band)	-
15.4	16.4	322	-
17.9	13.1	344	2.6
19.2	10.5	344	-
21.5	12.6	368	3.6
23.8	9.0	313	-
28.5	4.4	322	2.3
31.0	5.6	350	2.2

This value is lower than that obtained for sample A7, which possesses
longer PEO grafts.

The optical microscopic study undertaken on these systems proved
to be particularly fruitful. Systems A4 display most of the microscopic textures so far encountered in the smectic A phases of thermotropic liquid crystals or lyotropic systems (soaps, small nonionic
surfactants...). Classical focal conic, fan-shaped and mosaic textures,
as well as "oily streaks" and "batonnets" are easily observed. An
example of a fan-shaped texture is given in fig. 5. In this texture,
derived of the focal conic, the ellipses are not recognizable since
they lie in planes perpendicular to the film and are arranged along
the edges of the fan-like but the hyperbolae are visible and appear as
straight lines. Such well defined textures have not yet been observed
in amphiphilic copolymers. Moreover, we identified the recently dis-
covered parabolic focal conic (PFC) structure. This defect consisting
of polygonal arrays and described by Rosenblatt et al. [19] on a thermotropic smectic A liquid crystal was observed subsequently in systems
containing petroleum sulfonates [20] and lipid-water mixtures [21]. Our
observations are the first in systems containing polymeric emulsifiers.

In a smectic A phase, the molecules arrange themselves in two dimensional liquid layers which are easily curved but still of constant
thickness; these layers follow the well-known cyclides de Dupin [22],
with their associated singularities, the focal conics. Rosenblatt et
al [19], suggested that the PFC structure was a limiting case of the
focal conic defect in which the hyperbola and the ellipse are deformed
into a pair of confocal parabolae.

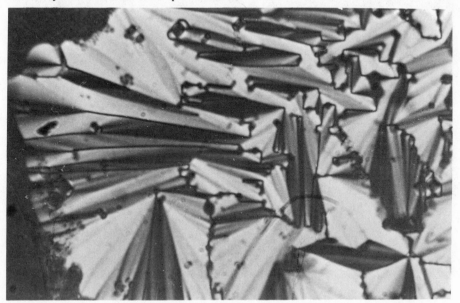

Fig. 5. Example of a fan-shaped texture observed between crossed
polarizers for sample A4 (G = 1000).

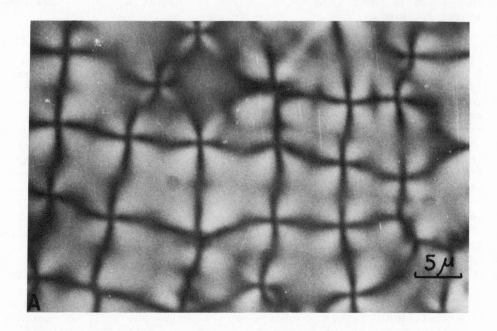

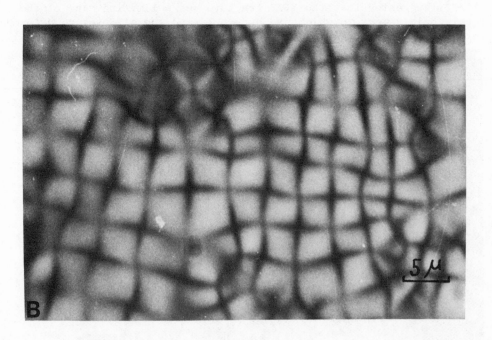

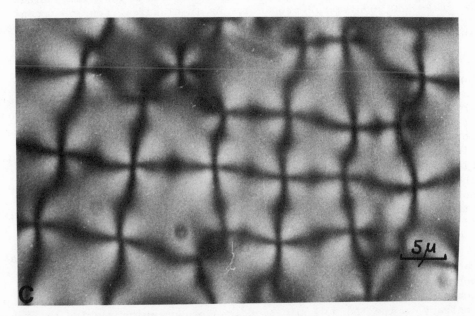

Fig. 6. Photomicrographs of the PFC structure observed for system
A4 (point P, fig. 1).
a) top plane,   b) mid-plane,   c) bottom plane of the capillary

Figure 6 shows three photomicrographs of the polygonal arrays
obtained when viewed between crossed polarizers. These three pictures
were taken by focusing the microscope on the top surface, the mid-
plane and the bottom surface of the capillary. They appear as three
related arrays composed of black intersecting lines. The corners of
the squares of the top surface are right above the centers of those of
the bottom surface. As for the middle cellular structure, located
half-way between the glass slides, its period is half that of the top
or the bottom, about 4μ. The parabolae intersect at the mid-height,
with their anchoring points on the top and bottom surfaces at the
corners of the squares.

The PFC structures that we observed for systems A4 form spontaneously in the capillary. Initially, the sample shows a rather weak
birefringence. After a short time the solution relaxes to a lower
energy state and an array of polygonal defects is produced, mainly
between the oily streaks which are formed. This polygonal structure
remains stable for a long period of time.

CONCLUSION

In this study, we identified the structures encountered in dif-

ferent parts of the phase diagram of the quaternary systems toluene/
water PS-PEO copolymer/2-propanol. As in classical four-component
systems, the structures of the monophasic domains depend strongly on
the surfactant/cosurfactant ratio.

The area I, characterized by a small value of this ratio (i.e.
copolymer/2-propanol), consists of mono or polymolecular normal
micelles (in the macromolecular sense of the word), swollen by a ternary solvent mixture of composition close to that of the external phase.
Inverted micelles which form in toluenic regions, i.e. in area II, are
obtained for higher copolymer concentrations and lower amounts of
alcohol. In some respects, these systems are analogous to nonionic
microemulsions. The birefringent area III must not be confused with
the microemulsion state and is completely different from the isotropic
solutions. This liquid-crystalline phase has an inverse cylindrical
structure or a lamellar structure depending on the chemical composition of the polymeric surfactant.

An interesting result is the experimental evidence of well characterized optical textures not observed previously on amphiphilic
copolymers. More specifically, we identified the parabolic focal
conic (PFC) defect which forms spontaneously in our lyotropic systems,
contrary to the thermotropic smectic A phases which require external
mechanical forces. These liquid-crystalline phases which associate
the fluidity of lyotropic systems and large dimensions of lamellae
should be particularly suitable to a study of defects in polymeric
compounds.

ACKNOWLEDGEMENTS

We would like to thank F. Debeauvais for helpful assistance in
the optical study and J. C. Wittmann for useful discussions. Our
thanks are also due to B. Lotz and A. Gonthier for much assistance in
the X-ray work.

REFERENCES

1. A. Skoulios and G. Finaz, J. Chim. Phys., 473 (1962)
2. F. M. Merrett, Trans. Far. Soc., 50, 759 (1954)
3. G. E. Molau, Block Polymers, S. L. Aggarwal, Plenum Press, New
    York, 79 (1970)
4. G. Riess, J. Nervo, D. Rogez, Polym. Prepr. Am. Chem. Soc., 18,
    329 (1977)
5. P. Marie and Y. Gallot, Cr. Acad. Sci., C, 284, 327 (1977)
6. J. Boutillier and F. Candau, Colloid and Polym. Sci., 257, 46
    (1979)
7. F. Ballet and F. Candau, Colloid and Polym. Sci. (submitted for
    publication)
8. F. Candau and J. C. Wittmann, Mol. Cryst. Liq. Cryst., 56, 171
    (1980)

9.   F. Candau, F. Afchar-Taromi and P. Rempp, Polymer, 18, 1253
     (1977)
10. J. Boutillier and F. Candau, Cr. Acad. Sci., 286 209 (1978)
11. Z. Tuzar and P. Kratochvil, Adv. in Colloid and Int., 6, 201
     (1976)
12. M. Hert, C. Strazielle and H. Benoit, Makromol. Chem., 171, 169
     (1973)
13. F. Candau, J. Boutillier, F. Tripier and J. C. Wittmann, Polymer,
     20, 1221 (1979)
     F. Candau, J. M. Guenet, J. Boutillier and Cl. Picot, Polymer,
     20, 1227 (1979)
     S. Candau, J. Boutillier and F. Candau, Polymer, 20, 1237 (1979)
14. L. M. Prince "Microemulsions", Acad. Press Inc. New-York (1977)
15. F. M. Menger and G. Saito, J. Amer. Chem. Soc., 100, 4376 (1978)
16. C. Kumar and D. Balasubramanian, J. Colloid and Interface Sci.,
     69, 271 (1979)
17. A. Skoulios, Adv. in Coll. and Int. Sci., 1, 79 (1967)
18. J. H. Schulman, R. Matalon and M. Cohen, Disc. Faraday Soc.,
     11, 117 (1951)
19. C. S. Rosenblatt, R. Pindak, N. A. Clark and R. B. Meyer, J.
     Physique, 38 1105 (1977)
20. W. J. Benton, E. W. Toor, C. A. Miller and T. Fort Ir., J.
     Physique, 40, 107 (1979)
21. S. A. Asher and P. S. Pershan., J. Physique, 40, 161 (1979)
22. G. Friedel, Ann. Phys., 2, 273 (1922).

Prof. P. Stenius: To what extent do the lipophilic layers in the
lamellar structures formed by the graft copolymers swell with toluene?

Dr F. Candau: The quasi-totality of the available toluene is presumably incorporated in the lipophilic layers, since toluene is a non-
solvent of the poly(ethylene oxide) sequences at room temperature.

Dr J. F. Holzwarth: What are the lifetimes and stability of the
structures you have shown?

Dr F. Candau: Because of the polymeric nature of the micellar
enveloppe, the interface is quite rigid and the lifetimes of the
micelles should be very large as compared to those of classical microemulsions formed with soaps. These polymeric systems are quite similar, as far as the stability is concerned, to biological systems such
as liposomes or vesicles.

Dr J. E. Crooks: Can you give an estimate of the diameter of the
spheres containing water in the classical microemulsion domain?

Dr F. Candau: Contrary to the case of systems I located in the upper
part of the phase diagram, the size of the inverted micelles of system
II is hard to determine. The main reasons are the fairly high copoly-

mer concentration and the difficulty in finding a procedure of dilution which does not modify the characteristics of the systems. However
an estimation is given by a photomicrograph after freeze fracturing,
which shows compact droplets with a diameter of about 200 Å.

Dr I. D. Robb: What are the parabolic curves you have shown and why
do they occur?

Dr F. Candau: The focal conics are defects frequently encountered in
the study of smectic phases by optical microscopy. The pair of focal
conics observed optically is generally formed of an ellipse and one
branch of an hyperbola around which the smectic sheets are curved and
fit "Dupin Cyclides", a family of equi-distant surfaces. The parabolic focal conic (PFC) structure I have shown is a limiting case of
the classical focal conic defect, the hyperbola and the ellipse being
deformed into a pair of confocal parabolae. The focal conic arrangement is the consequence of forces which prevent attainment of the
uniaxial planar texture (homeotropy) and is a configuration of minimum strain.

VISCOSITY AND CONDUCTIVITY OF MICROEMULSIONS

K. E. Bennett, J. C. Hatfield, H. T. Davis, C. W. Macosko
and L. E. Scriven
Department of Chemical Engineering and Materials Science
University of Minnesota
Minneapolis, Minnesota 55455

INTRODUCTION

Flooding with surfactant-based microemulsions is one of the
promising techniques for enhancing petroleum recovery from natural
deposits, or reservoirs[1]. By microemulsion we mean a thermodynamically stable, microstructured fluid phase of variable composition
that incorporates substantial amounts of oil, water and surfactants.
The phase behaviour, interfacial tensions, and rheological properties
of a microemulsion formulation are among the primary determinants of
the potential success of a microemulsion flood. Because the number
of equilibrium phases, their volumes and their appearances are easier
to measure and observe than phase compositions, viscosities and interfacial tensions, there is obvious interest in understanding the relationship between the phase counts, volumes and appearances and the
other physical properties of microemulsions[2,3].

To recover oil, a microemulsion has to have ultralow tensions,
$\gamma_{O/M}$ and $\gamma_{M/W}$ against oil-rich and water-rich phases, respectively.
The optimal salinity has been defined[3] as the salinity at which
these tensions are equal (see Fig. 1). Tension measurements are
rather time-consuming and can be quite tedious; and since hundreds of
samples may be involved in surfactant screening tests, it was an
important discovery[3] that optimal salinity is almost the same as
the salinity of equal oil and water volume uptake by the microemulsion
phase. A salinity scan is perhaps the method most frequently used to
find the salinity of equal volume uptake for a candidate surfactant
formulation. Typical salinity scans are illustrated in Figs. 1 and 2
for mixtures containing about equal amounts of oil and water. As
salinity increases from left to right, the surfactant-rich, or microemulsion, phase is first the brine-rich, water-continuous, lower phase

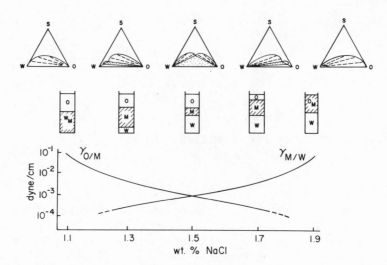

Fig. 1. Schematic of a typical microemulsion salinity scan showing the progression of phase diagrams, phase volumes and interfacial tensions.

in a two-phase system ($\underline{2}$); then the middle phase solubilizing significant amounts of oil and brine in a three-phase system (3); and finally an oil-rich, oil-continuous, upper phase in a two-phase system ($\overline{2}$). The mnemonic $\underline{2}$-3-$\overline{2}$ notation, introduced by Knickerbocker et al.[4], gives the number of equilibrium phases and the location of the surfactant-rich one.

Because the viscosity is also an important factor in the ability of microemulsion to recover oil, it is necessary either to measure viscosities of the numerous samples being evaluated or to discover relationships between the viscosity and the more easily measured phase counts, volumes and appearances.

The search for such relationships is part of the motivation for the work presented here. We report extensive measurements of microemulsion viscosity and electrical conductivity along with phase counts, opacity and volume uptake of oil and brine in the microemulsion; salinity and hydrocarbon chain length are varied, and both pure and commercial alkyl aryl sulfonate surfactants are used. A deeper goal of our research is to try to identify the microstructures present in microemulsion and relate these to the physical properties. Although there is general agreement that at low salinity the lower phase microemulsion ($\underline{2}$) is a water-continuous solution of oil-swollen micelles and that at high salinity the upper phase microemulsion ($\overline{2}$) is

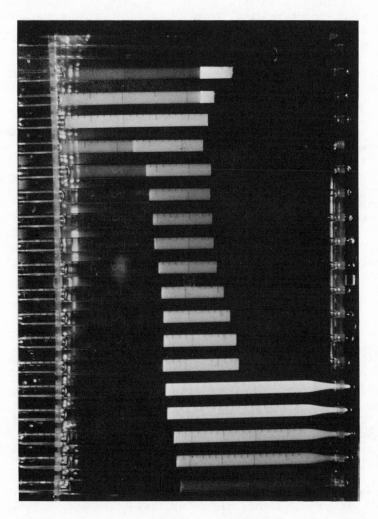

1.0 1.4 1.6 1.8 1.9 2.0 2.1 2.2 2.3 2.5 2.6 2.8 2.9 3.0 3.2 3.4 3.6 4.0

Fig. 2. Photograph of the TRS 10–80/tAA/nC$_{14}$ salinity scan at 25 °C. From left to right the salinities, in g NaCl/100 cm^3 brine

probably an oil-continuous solution of water-swollen inverted micelles, some question persists as to the microstructure at intermediate salinities, where microemulsion is able to take up substantial amounts (even equal amounts) of both water and oil. It has been conjectured[5] that in this intermediate region a microemulsion is a submicroscopically bicontinuous interspersion, i.e., there are sample spanning paths through both oil-rich and water-rich materials in the microemulsion. The role of surfactant is to separate the oil-rich and water-rich parts of the microstructure in a thermodynamically stable way, which probably involves a surfactant-rich, multiply-connected, sheet-like region that confers topological order.

The qualitative patterns of phase behaviour of microemulsion have been mimicked by a statistical mechanical model[6,7] based on the assumption that microemulsion is a random interspersion of water and oil separated by surfactant monolayers. A disordered interspersion of this type is expected, as outlined in the Discussion, to exhibit percolative behaviour and to have a bicontinuous structure over a wide range of oil-water ratios.

The observed conductivity behaviour of microemulsion has, in fact, been interpreted previously by one of us[8] and by others[9,10] in terms of percolation theory. Recently published self-diffusion studies[11] provide further evidence for bicontinuous structures. The possibility of explaining the viscosity as well as the conductivity behaviour of a microemulsion in terms of percolation concepts will be addressed in the Discussion.

EXPERIMENTAL

The pure surfactant used in this study was sodium 4-(1-heptylnonyl)benzenesulfonate (SHBS), known elsewhere as SPHS[12] or as Texas No. 1.[13,14]. It was synthesized at the University of Texas under a Department of Energy contract to W. H. Wade and R. S. Schechter. The commercial surfactant used was Witco Chemical Company's TRS 10-80. Both surfactants were used as received. The tertiary amyl alcohol (tAA), isobutyl alcohol (iBA) and straight chain n-alkanes (nC_8, nC_{10}, and nC_{14}) used were at least 98% pure and were obtained from Aldrich Chemical, Fischer Scientific, Eastman Kodak, or Phillips Petroleum.

All brine solutions were made with dried, reagent-grade NaCl (Fischer Scientific) and doubly-distilled, deionized water; concentrations are expressed in g NaCl/100 cm^3 solution. Two surfactant-alcohol-oil stock solutions were used: the one contained 0.325g SHBS, 0.65g iBA and 10ml n-alkane; the other contained 0.40g TRS 10-80, 0.20g tAA and 10ml n-alkane. Salinity scans are indexed by giving the surfactant/alcohol/n-alkane combination used. The samples were prepared by mixing equal volumes of brine and surfactant-alcohol-oil stock solution and were sealed inside 5ml Corning Disposable Serologi-

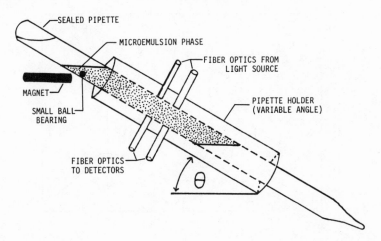

Fig. 3.   Schematic of the multiphase rolling ball viscometer (from
Bennett et al[15]).

cal Pipets (which came marked in 0.1 ml increments). The sample preparation, equilibration and viewing procedures are described in detail
elsewhere[14]. The microemulsion opacity data presented here are
qualitative measurements by direct visual observation.

The viscosity of each microemulsion phase was measured using the
multiphase rolling ball viscometer (Fig. 3) developed by Bennett et
al[15], in which a 1mm diameter stainless steel ball-bearing rolls
through the liquid phase of interest. As it travels past each of the
two fiber optic cables, the ball interrupts a light beam, producing
a voltage pulse at the corresponding detector. The travel time
between the two voltage pulses is measured electronically and is
related to liquid viscosity by calibration with Newtonian oils of
known viscosity. All reported viscosities are the average of at
least 5 measurements. Error bars, for ± 2 standard deviations (95%
confidence interval), are given for errors greater than the size of
the data points.

Electrical conductivity was measured in two different apparatuses
three years apart. The earlier data[8] (shown as dots in Figs. 4b,
5b and 6b) were taken at 23°C using a Jones-type conductivity cell and
a hand-balanced a.c. conductance bridge. Recently data (shown as
open circles in Figs. 5b, 6b and 10) were obtained at 25°C using the
same cell but with a Brinkmann E518 direct-indicating conductometer,
the sensitivity of which is several orders of magnitude greater than
that of the a.c. conductance bridge. Samples were equilibrated for
at least 5 days at the same temperature as the conductivity cell.

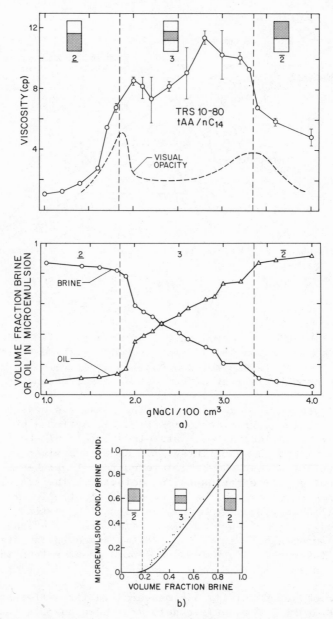

Fig. 4. TRS 10-80/tAA/nC_14 brine salinity scan. All data except where noted below were taken at 25°C. a) Microemulsion viscosity, microemulsion opacity (qualitative) and volume fraction of brine or oil in the microemulsion versus salinity in g NaCl/100 cm³ brine. Error bars, for ±2 standard deviations (95% confidence interval), are given for viscosity errors greater than the size of the data points. The vertical dashed lines mark the salinities at the 2-3 and 3-2̄ phase transitions.

Fig. 4b) Ratio of the electrical conductivity of microemulsion to the electrical conductivity of brine used to make the sample versus volume fraction of brine; increasing volume fraction corresponds to decreasing salinity. The vertical dashed lines mark the volume fractions at the $\overline{2}$-3 and 3-$\underline{2}$ transitions. The solid curve is the theoretical prediction of Winterfeld[19]. The dots are data for samples at 23°C.

Samples were transferred to the conductivity cell at approximately $3cm^3/sec$ through a 13 gauge needle. Conductivity was recorded after it remained constant for at least 4 minutes.

The volume fraction of oil or brine in the microemulsion phase was estimated from the observed equilibrium phase volumes and the overall composition, on the assumptions that the alcohol was in the same phase as the surfactant and that negligible brine and oil were solubilized by the excess oil and brine phases, respectively. Thus, the volume of brine or oil in the microemulsion equaled the total in the sample less the volume of the appropriate excess phase.

RESULTS

Fig. 2 is a photograph of the TRS 10-80/tAA/nC_{14} salinity scan. As salinity increases, the opacity of the microemulsion increases up to the 2-3 transition, decreases rapidly, peaks again at the 3-$\overline{2}$ transition and then decreases steadily. The volume of the microemulsion phase also has maxima occurring at the 2-3 and 3-$\overline{2}$ transitions in a salinity scan. The viscosity of the microemulsion phase is plotted versus salinity in Fig. 4a; the vertical dashed lines mark the salinities for the 2-3 and 3-$\overline{2}$ transitions. There are two peaks in microemulsion viscosity, apparently related to the two peaks in opacity and to the two phase transitions. Reed and Healy[3] observed similar viscosity peaks at the 2-3 and 3-$\overline{2}$ transitions. Their data led them to suggest that microemulsion undergoes a microstructural transition at each viscosity peak and that these peaks occur at the 2-3 and 3-$\overline{2}$ transitions. However, viscosity peaks and phase transitions do not coincide in all the systems reported here.

The plot of volume fraction of brine or oil solubilized in the microemulsion (Fig. 4a) gives no indication of where the viscosity peaks occur. However, near optimal salinity, as measured by equal volume uptake of oil and brine into the microemulsion, the viscosity is a local minimum. Fig. 4b gives the ratio of the electrical conductivity of microemulsion to the electrical conductivity of the brine as a function of volume fraction of the brine in the microemulsion. Note that increasing volume fraction brine corresponds to decreasing salinity. The solid curve is a theoretical result which is discussed below. The conductivity ratio varies smoothly over the entire 2-3-$\overline{2}$ scan and does not suggest any of the features of the viscosity data. Reed and Healy[3] also noted this lack of correlation.

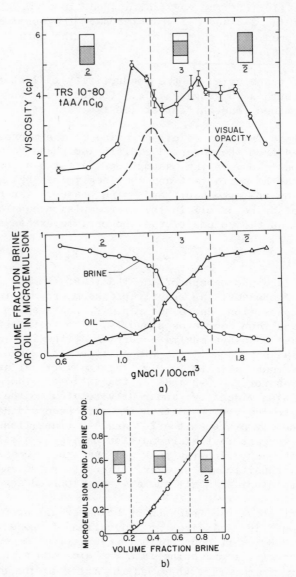

Fig. 5.   TRS 10-80/tAA/nC$_{10}$ salinity scan (see caption, Fig. 4). The
dots and open circles in b) are conductivity ratio data of samples at
23°C and 25°C, respectively.

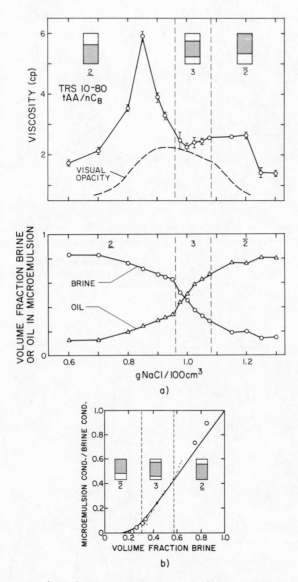

Fig. 6.   TRS 10-80/tAA/nC$_8$ salinity scan (see caption, Fig. 4).   The dots and open circles in b) are conductivity ratio data of samples at 23°C and 25°C, respectively.

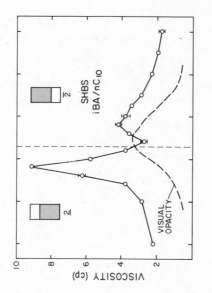

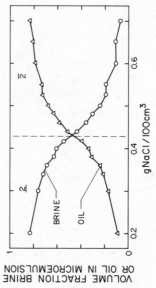

Fig. 8. SHBS/iBA/nC$_{10}$ salinity scan (see caption, Fig. 4a). Vertical dashed line marks the salinity at the 2-$\overline{2}$ transition.

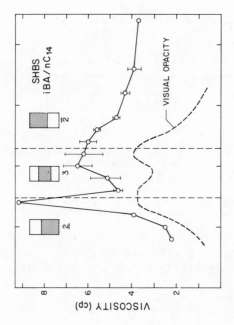

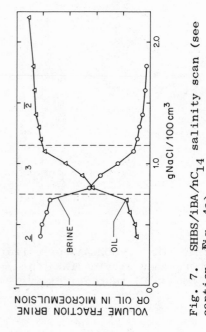

Fig. 7. SHBS/iBA/nC$_{14}$ salinity scan (see caption, Fig. 4a).

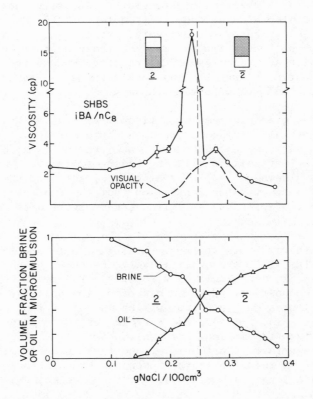

Fig. 9.   SHBS/iBA/**nC**$_8$ salinity scan (see captions, Figs. 4a and 8).

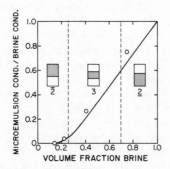

Fig. 10.   SHBS/iBA/nC$_{12}$ salinity scan.   Conductivity ratios for samples at 25°C (see caption, Fig. 4b).

Figs. 5 and 6 show the microemulsion viscosity, opacity, volume fraction and electrical conductivity data for the TRS 10–80/tAA/nC$_{10}$ and nC$_8$ salinity scans, respectively. As in Fig. 4, the viscosity in each scan goes through two maxima, and these do not consistently correlate with any features of the opacity, volume fraction or electrical conductivity curves. The local minimum in the viscosity curves occurs near equal volume uptake, however.

Figs. 7–9 give microemulsion viscosity, opacity and volume fraction data for salinity scans using the pure surfactant SHBS, the alcohol iBA and the n-alkanes nC$_{14}$, nC$_{10}$ and nC$_8$. With nC$_{10}$ and nC$_8$ there is a 2-$\overline{2}$ transition with increasing salinity. This indicates, as detailed elsewhere[14], that at optimal salinity the middle phase has a lower surfactant concentration that the concentration at the mixing point. Fig. 10 shows limited conductivity data for the SHBS/iBA/nC$_{12}$ salinity scan.

The data with both the pure surfactant SHBS and the commercial surfactant TRS 10–80 are qualitatively the same. Each salinity scan has two peaks in microemulsion viscosity. The peaks coincide neither with phase boundaries, peaks in microemulsion opacity, nor with any apparent features of the volume uptake and electrical conductivity curves. There is, however, one correlation for the systems studied here: the viscosity minimum between the two peaks always occurs near equal volume uptake. Furthermore, the first peak in microemulsion viscosity grows relative to the second as hydrocarbons of shorter and shorter chain length are mixed with either surfactant.

DISCUSSION

Such macroscopic properties of microemulsion as viscosity, interfacial tensions, electrical conductivity and phase behaviour must be related to fluid microstructures. Several structures for microemulsion have been proposed including spherical micelles, inverted micelles, and mixtures thereof[16]; lamellar, tubular and globular structures[16]; and equilibrium bicontinuous structures[5]. It has been suggested[8–10] that the electrical conductivity of microemulsion exhibits percolative behaviour expected of a disordered interspersion capable of bicontinuous structures. This possibility can be examined in terms of the model interspersion introduced by Talmon and Prager[6] to pursue the thermodynamic consequences of the bicontinuous hypothesis. They have represented microemulsion as a random interspersion of oil and water in Voronoi polyhedra, the surfactant lying between oil and water regions and having negligible volume. The Voronoi polyhedra (Fig. 11) are formed by randomly distributing points in space, drawing bisecting planes between points, and forming the edges of the polyhedra faces from intersecting planes so as to divide space into convex polyhedra[17]. As mentioned above, the model of Talmon and Prager predicts sequences of ternary phase diagrams that are qualitatively similar to those of microemulsion systems[6,7].

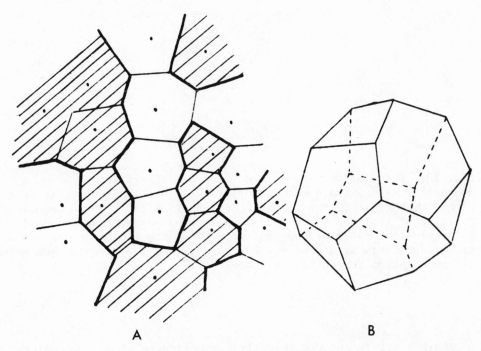

A   B

Fig. 11. A Voronoi representation of a bicontinuous microemulsion.
a) Two dimensional example. Shaded regions are occupied by oil-like
material, unshaded regions by water-like material; heavy lines
indicate the surfactant layer. b) Typical Voronoi polyhedron. From
Talmon and Prager[6].

The percolative behaviour of a random interspersion especially
pertinent to the present paper is illustrated in Fig. 12. ϕ denotes
the volume fraction of one of the materials, say the water, of the
interspersion. If the volume fraction of water is less than the
"percolation threshold" ϕ_c of the water, then the oil phase is
continuous and all the water is isolated, i.e., it is surrounded by
oil. For volume fractions of water above the percolation threshold
ϕ_c of the water, some of the water becomes sample-spanning, i.e.,
there exists a continuous path of water reaching from one side of the
sample to the other. The total volume fraction ϕ of water is the sum
of the fraction ϕ^I of isolated water and the fraction ϕ^A of continuous
water, shown as solid curves in Fig. 12. Since oil and water are
treated symmetrically in the model, the isolated and continuous oil
fractions are curves (dashed) similar to ϕ^I and ϕ^A, increasing oil
fraction $(1-\phi)$ being read from right to left in Fig. 12. For volume
fractions of water lying between ϕ_c and $1-\phi_c$ (shaded region), the
random interspersion is bicontinuous, finite fractions of both water
and oil forming sample-spanning paths.

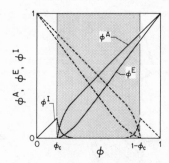

Fig. 12.   Percolative behaviour of a random interspersion of
conductor, water, and nonconductor, oil. ϕ denotes the volume fraction of water, (1-ϕ) the volume fraction of oil; ϕ^I and ϕ^A denote the
fraction of isolated water and of continuous water, respectively;
ϕ^E denotes the ratio of the conductivity of the random interspersion
to the conductivity of the water phase; ϕ_c and 1-ϕ_c are the water and
oil percolation thresholds, respectively.

        Since oil is not electrically conducting, a disordered inter-
spersion will have zero conductivity when the water fraction falls
below its percolation threshold ϕ_c.   Slightly above the percolation
threshold the conductivity will still be relatively small because the
conducting channels of water are rather tortuous.   The quantity ϕ^E
shown in Fig. 12 denotes the ratio of the conductivity of the random
interspersion to the conductivity of the conducting phase of the
interspersion.   The qualitative shape of the curve of ϕ^E versus ϕ
shown in Fig. 12 has been verified in a number of computer simula-
tions[18,19].   There is an almost linear region (where the effective
medium approximation[20], $\phi^E \approx \frac{3}{2}\phi - \frac{1}{2}$, is roughly obeyed) and a
non-linear region near the percolation threshold where ϕ^E is propor-
tional to $(\phi - \phi_c)^\upsilon$, υ being of the order of 1.6.[18].

        Winterfeld[19] has computed ϕ^E for the random interspersion
generated with the Voronoi polyhedra. He estimated the percolation
threshold to be ϕ_c = 0.16.   His results are the solid curve drawn
Figs. 4b, 5b, 6b and 10 containing the conductivity data on the various microemulsions.   These predictions mimic surprisingly well the
experimental observations.   Although this is the first time microemulsion conductivity results have been compared directly with conductivities predicted with the random Voronoi interspersion, it has been
remarked before[9,10] that, near the percolation threshold, the shape
of the curve of relative conductivity ϕ^E versus volume fraction of
water is of the form predicted by percolation theory, although
Lagües[9b] has argued that dynamical effects lead to percolation
exponents different from those predicted by static models.

For volume fractions of brine above 0.3, the experimental conductivity ratios are linear in volume fraction with a least-squares fit
of the data giving slopes of 1.24, 1.33, 1.55, and 1.43 and intercepts
of -0.24, -0.32, -0.44 and -0.30 for Figs. 4b, 5b, 6b and 10, respectively. The data in Figs. 6b and 10 extrapolate to conductivity ratios
greater than the volume fraction ϕ, presumably because the conductivity
of the ionic surfactant becomes important at low salinities.

We believe the qualitative agreement between the conductivity of
microemulsion and the random Voronoi interspersion is significant and
argues strongly for the existence of bicontinuous microstructures in
microemulsion under certain conditions. However, the quantitative
agreement may be fortuitous. The interfaces between water and oil
regions are probably graded zones rather than even near discontinui-
ties. It is certainly unlikely that interfaces in the real system
have the kind of angularity implied by the Voronoi-construct or that
the surfactant has negligible volume. Also, it is unlikely that
water and oil behave equivalently or that the interspersion is totally
random. Local interactions between surfactant molecules and other
components of microemulsion surely create correlations biasing the
morphology of the interspersion, e.g., through preferred states of
curvature of surfactant-rich zones[5]. Also, unlike the model, microemulsion is a dynamical system: the interspersion morphology must
change continuously under thermal fluctuations, paths being continuously broken and mended and isolates created and destroyed (by coales-
cing with continuous material)[5,8]. As mentioned above, it has
indeed been suggested[9b] that the qualitative aspects of the behaviour of ϕ^E in microemulsions reflects dynamical effects. That the
making and breaking of any existing local microstructure is relatively
easy (energetically) is implied by the relatively low viscosities of
microemulsion compared to liquid crystals or gels, for example.

It is possible, however, that all these factors merely distort
somewhat the shapes of the curves, ϕ^I, ϕ^A, and ϕ^E, leaving intact
their qualitative structure and percolative nature. The agreement
between microemulsion conductivity and predictions of the Voronoi
interspersion suggests that this is the case.

The fact that the conductivity does not reflect the viscosity
undulations observed in microemulsion represents further support for
a bicontinuous structure. The charge carriers presumably move through
water channels, the viscosity of which is relatively unaffected by
the local morphology of the interspersion. Shear of the microemulsion,
on the other hand, involves the cutting across or the deforming of
local microstructures and therefore can be expected to give a viscosity that changes with the changing oil-water distributions in the
interspersion. The viscosity behaviour anticipated from the picture
of a microemulsion as a random interspersion is as follows. If one
phase is discontinuous ($\phi < \phi_c$ or $\phi > 1 - \phi_c$ in Fig. 12), we expect,
from known behaviour of dispersions, the viscosity to increase with

increasing volume fraction of the discontinuous phase. At the percolation threshold, the random interspersion undergoes a microstructural
transition. The mechanism of momentum transfer under shear must
change at this point. In the bicontinuous region shear must involve
breaking and remending local microstructures, i.e., topological
changes. Outside the bicontinuous region, shear need not break the
discontinuous structures-- it may simply rotate or deform them. Thus,
we might expect to see sharp changes in the viscosity trends with
salinity at the water and oil percolation thresholds.

In support of this expectation, the high salinity (oil-rich
microemulsion) break in viscosity observed in a salinity scan occurs
quite close (Figs. 5 and 6) to the water percolation threshold located
by the conductivity data. We conjecture that the low salinity (water-
rich microemulsion) peak in viscosity occurs at the oil percolation
threshold. This hypothesis can be tested by locating the oil percolation threshold by measuring, as did Lindman et al.[11] for a different
microemulsion, the diffusivity of a solute soluble in oil but not in
water.

If the oil-like and brine-like regions in a bicontinuous microstructure were equivalent, as in the Voronoi model, the viscosity at
equal volume uptake of oil and brine would, from symmetry, be either
a local maximum or a local minimum. For the systems studied here a
local minimum occurs near equal volume uptake.

The two peaks in viscosity with increasing salinity imply the
existence of at least three microstructural regimes, one before, one
between, and one after the two peaks. The coincidence of the start
of one viscosity peak with the conductivity percolation threshold
argues that the peaks are indicative of the transition from mono- to
bicontinuous microstructures.

What we cannot explain at present is why the viscosity would
decrease as the microstructure becomes increasingly bicontinuous,
unless the resistance itself of the material to topological change
falls. Certainly, if the microstructure were ordered, as in a liquid
crystal, or relatively difficult to break, as in a gel, then the
viscosity might be expected to increase with increasing bicontinuity.
Further research on this problem is needed.

SUMMARY

For the systems studied here, microemulsion viscosity goes
through two maxima as salinity increases. The viscosity peaks do not
correlate with phase boundaries, peaks in microemulsion opacity, nor
with any apparent features of the volume uptake curves. However, the
local viscosity minimum does correspond closely to equal volume uptake
of oil and brine into the microemulsion. The data with both the pure
surfactant SHBS and the commercial surfactant TRS 10-80 are qualita-

tively the same, implying that our conclusions are not limited to the particular systems studied. It should be noted, however, that contrary to the results of Reed and Healy[3] and all those reported here, Salter[21], using several different commercial surfactants, observed only single peaks in microemulsion viscosity with increasing salinity. The reasons for this different behaviour are not yet clear.

Electrical conductivity data exhibit a percolation threshold in brine volume fraction and agree remarkably well with predictions based on a model for a random interspersion of conducting and non-conducting material. The model predicts three structural regimes: discontinuous oil in brine, bicontinuous oil and brine, and discontinuous brine in oil. The discrete oil and brine of the model can be interpreted as oil-like and brine-like regions in the thermodynamically stable microstructure of a microemulsion. The observed double viscosity peak in a salinity scan also implies three microstructural regimes for microemulsion. One break in the viscosity versus salinity curve occurs near the brine percolation threshold as determined by electrical conductivity; presumably the second break is related to the oil percolation threshold.

We conjecture that of the continuous range of possibilities discussed elsewhere,[5,16], the microstructures in the systems studied here progress with increasing salinity from a solution of swollen micelles to a bicontinuous microstructure rich in water to a bicontinuous microstructure rich in oil to a solution of swollen inverted micelles.

ACKNOWLEDGEMENT

We are grateful to the Department of Energy for financial support of this work.

REFERENCES

1. W. B. Gogarty, J. Pet. Tech., $\underline{28}$, 93 (1976).
2. M. L. Robbins, in "Micellization, Solubilization and Microemulsions," ed. K. L. Mittal (Plenum Press, New York, 1977) 713-744; P. D. Fleming, III and J. E. Vinatieri, AIChe J., $\underline{25}$, 493 (1979); P. D. Fleming, III, J. E. Vinatieri and G. R. Glinsmann, J. Phys. Chem., $\underline{84}$, 1526 (1980).
3. R. L. Reed and R. N. Healy, in "Improved Oil Recovery by Surfactant and Polymer Flooding," eds. D. O. Shah and R. S. Schechter (Academic Press, New York, 1977) 383-437.
4. B. M. Knickerbocker, C. V. Pesheck, L. E. Scriven and H. T. Davis, J. Phys. Chem., $\underline{83}$, 1984 (1979).
5. L. E. Scriven, Nature, $\underline{263}$, 123 (1976); L. E. Scriven, in "Micellization, Solubilization, and Microemulsions," Vol. 2, ed. K. L. Mittal (Plenum Press, New York, 1977) 877-893.
6. Y. Talmon and S. Prager, Nature, $\underline{267}$, 333 (1977); J. Chem. Phys., $\underline{69}$, 2984 (1978).

7. H. T. Davis and L. E. Scriven, SPE 9278, presented at the 55th
    Annual Fall Meeting of the Soc. Pet. Eng., Dallas, Texas (Sept.
    21-24, 1980).
8. J. C. Hatfield, Ph.D. Thesis (University of Minnesota, 1978).
9. (a) M. Laguës, R. Ober and C. Taupin, J. Physique Lett., 39, L48
        (1978).
    (b) M. Laguës, J. Physique Lett., 40, L331 (1979).
    (c) M. Dvolaitzky, M. Laguës, J. P. Le Pesant, R. Ober,
        C. Sauterey and C. Taupin, J. Phys. Chem. 84, 1532 (1980).
10. B. Lagourette, J. Peyrelasse, C. Boned and M. Clausse, Nature,
    281, 60 (1979).
11. B. Lindman, N. Kamenka, T. Kathopoulis, B. Brun and P. Nilsson,
    J. Phys. Chem., 84, 2485 (1980).
12. E. I. Franses, J. E. Puig, Y. Talmon, W. G. Miller, L. E. Scriven
    and H. T. Davis, J. Phys. Chem., 84, 1547 (1980).
13. See, for example, J. E. Puig, E. I. Franses, Y. Talmon,
    H. T. Davis, W. G. Miller and L. E. Scriven, SPE 9349, presented
    at the 55th Annual Fall Meeting of the Soc. Pet. Eng., Dallas,
    Texas (Sept. 21-24, 1980).
14. K. E. Bennett, C. H. K. Phelps, H. T. Davis and L. E. Scriven,
    SPE 9351, presented at the 55th Annual Fall Meeting of the Soc.
    Pet. Eng., Dallas, Texas (Sept. 21-24, 1980).
15. K. E. Bennett, H. T. Davis, C. W. Macosko and L. E. Scriven,
    manuscript to be submitted to the AIChE J.
16. P. A. Winsor, Chem. Rev., 68, 1(1968); P. A. Winsor, in Liquid
    Crystals and Plastic Crystals, Vol. 1, eds. G. W. Gray and
    P. A. Winsor, (Ellis Horwood Ltd., Chichester, 1974), 199-
    287.
17. G. Voronoi, J. reine angew. Math., 134, 198 (1908).
18. S. Kirkpatrick, Rev. Mod. Phys., 45, 574 (1973).
19. P. W. Winterfeld, Ph.D. Thesis (University of Minnesota, 1981).
20. R. Landauer, J. Appl. Phys., 23, 779 (1952).
21. S. J. Salter, SPE 6843, presented at the 52nd Annual Fall Meeting
    of the Soc. Pet. Eng., Denver, Colorado (Oct. 9-12, 1977);
    private communication.

DISCUSSION

Prof. P. Stenius: We have found viscosity maxima in microemulsions,
containing roughly equal amounts of water and oil, which are similar
to those reported here. However, they cannot be correlated with the
number of phases that are in equilibrium with the microemulsion,
except in the sense that the three-phase regions often occur when
the O/W ratio is about 1.

Prof. H. T. Davis: One of the conclusions of our paper is that the
viscosity maxima do not correlate with the number of phases.

Dr E. Dickinson: It is supposed that the bicontinuous interspersion
is bounded by water-continuous and oil-continuous micellar solutions
at low and high oil concentrations respectively. In the extreme

regions are the viscosity results consistent with what one might
expect on the basis of a simple hard-sphere model?

Prof. H. T. Davis: The viscosity increases with volume fraction of
the discontinuous phase in qualitative, but not quantitative agreement
with the predictions of a hard-sphere model.

Dr F. T. Hesselink: Are the sharpness of the viscosity peaks related
to the polydispersity of the surfactants used?

Prof. H. T. Davis: Perhaps. However, the low-salinity peak, which
seems to be always the sharpest with both pure and commercial surfactant, is quite sharp in at least one instance (see Fig. 6) with the
commercial surfactant TRS 10-80. Comparison of Figs.4-6 shows that
the sharpness can be controlled by simply varying the hydrocarbon in
the microemulsion.

Prof. H. F. Eicke: Did the authors observe no discontinuity in proceeding from the transparent, low-viscous hydrocarbon solution phase
(= so-called microemulsion domain) to the so-called bi-continuous
state? Did the bicontinuous state appear turbid? Could the percolation threshold be interpreted as a "phase transition" from the solution phase to the bicontinuous state?

Prof. H. T. Davis: One can perhaps define a continuity transition,
detected as percolation thresholds of conductivity and diffusion and
perhaps as viscosity peaks, but not as a phase transition. All of
the samples, both in the presumably bicontinuous and mono-continuous
regimes, appeared homogeneous; most samples scattered light as indicated by the opacity curves given for each salinity scan. From the
way you pose the question I do not think we agree on the definition
of microemulsion. We consider the bicontinuous state to be microemulsion also.

Prof. B. Lindman: You have obtained very nice data on the detailed
concentration dependence of microemulsion viscosity. A striking
general observation seems to be the rather low viscosities. For isotropic surfactant solutions known to contain extended aggregates such
as rod micelles (concentrated CTAB solution, etc.) or cubic liquid
crystals, the viscosities are up to orders of magnitude higher than
you observe. This might suggest that your microemulsions do not contain extended structures. Do you think this is a reasonable argument?

Prof. H. T. Davis: It is indeed striking that the viscosity is rather
low in the regions interpreted as bicontinuous. The structures may be
considerably diffuse, as Winsor[16] reasoned and we have discussed
elsewhere[5], and they are certainly dynamical in nature. Thus, the
bicontinuous arrangement seems unlikely to exist as a static, extended
structure. It certainly follows from the viscosity data that the
microstructures are easily broken and mended (no strongly non-

Newtonian behaviour was observed with the rolling ball viscometer).

Prof. B. Lemanceau: In the case of TRS 10-80 as surfactant the result
are difficult to interpret, as it is not a pure, homogeneous compound.
How does this affect the results and how do the constituents partition
between the various phases?

Prof. H. T. Davis: We deliberately practice the strategy of studying
the scientifically defined pure surfactant and the practically significant mixed surfactant in parallel. Our data indicate that the TRS
10-80 behaves qualitatively the same in these studies as does the pure
surfactant SHBS. We did not chemically analyze phase compositions.

STRUCTURAL AND SOLUBILIZATION PROPERTIES OF NONIONIC SURFACTANTS

A COMPARATIVE STUDY OF TWO HOMOLOGOUS SERIES

G. Mathis[+], J. C. Ravey[++] and M. Buzier[++]

[+] Laboratoire de Chimie Physique Organique
[++] Laboratoire de Biophysique Moléculaire
E.R.A. C.N.R.S., C.O. No. 140
54037 Nancy Cedex, France

INTRODUCTION

These last years the nonionic surfactants have attracted much interest. Despite that fact, and due to the tremendous number of possible investigations, the properties of systems containing nonionic surfactants are far to be well understood at the present time.

The systematic investigations of the phase behaviours have been recently initiated by Shinoda and Friberg[1-5], where the effect of various additives and of the temperature have been described for some particular systems.

Although the structural determinations on aqueous isotropic solutions of nonionic surfactants have been undertaken a few decades ago (by light scattering, X-ray scattering, ultra-centrifugation, NMR, osmometry, etc...)[6-12], most of the structural studies on oil/water (brine)/surfactant systems are very recent and may use other or very sophisticated techniques (pulsed NMR, neutron scattering, conductivity and dielectric measurements, etc...)[13-14]. However the results are far from coherent and definitive. So it remains much to be done, both in the phase stability and the structural investigations of such systems.

As a small contribution, the present paper concerns some studies on systems with nonionic surfactants which are linear polyoxyethylene alcohols: they differ by their hydrophobic parts which are either hydrogenated or fluorinated.

Indeed we are especially interested in the solubilization of fluorocarbons in water thanks to fluorinated surfactants.

Some results of a comparative study of their properties will be presented here, related to the water-oil solubilization properties, and to the structures of the micellar aggregates in the isotropic phases, which depend on the chemical nature of the surfactant and oil molecules, the salinity and the temperature. However most of the results concern the hydrogenated surfactants.

Given the lack of work on fluorinated surfactants, the interest of such a comparative study rests on the similitude of their behaviour with those of the hydrogenated homologous which are much better known It should be very useful to be able to extrapolate the properties of the fluorinated systems from those of the hydrogenated ones.

MATERIALS

A description of the molecules used in our study is given in Table I. For the hydrogenated systems, the number of oxyethylene groups is between 4 and 7, and the alkyl chain is a C_{10} or C_{12} one. The oils may be heptane, decane, hexadecane, cyclohexane and benzene. Three salts have been added: sodium carbonate, sodium chloride and calcium chloride, with concentrations less than 200 g/1. Both pure and technical grade surfactants have been studied, but not systematically.

In the homologous fluorinated surfactants, there are 6 to 7 carbons in the hydrophobic chain, and 2 or 11 to 14 oxyethylene groups Three fluorocarbons were also used. Most of the fluorinated compounds are pilot plant preparations supplied by P.C.U.K., and were obtained by condensation of ethylene oxide on a fluorinated alcohol. Thus the oxyethylene numbers are only mean values centred at 14 and 11.

RESULTS

1) Binary Mixtures in Water or in Oil

(a) The hydrogenated nonionic surfactants in water have a low value of the C.M.C., as it is well known[15]. In water, the C.M.C. decreases for increasing values of the temperature and of the salinity and for decreasing values of the H.L.B.; of course the larger the aggregation number the lower the C.M.C. is.

The properties of the surfactants in apolar media are much less known[14-16]. The partial results summarized below will be discussed in detail elsewhere. They have been obtained from some of our latest neutron scattering measurements.

For sufficiently apolar media, like decane, a critical concentration can also be evidenced, as can be seen by the curves of the neu-

Table 1

SURFACTANT	OIL	SALT	TEMPERATURE
Hydrogenated Systems			
$C_N H_{2N+1}(OC_2H_4)_M OH$	C_7H_{16}	Na_2CO_3	
N = 10 - 12	$C_{10}H_{22}$	Na Cl	50–90°C
M = 4 - 7	$C_{16}H_{34}$	Ca Cl$_2$	
(HLB = 10 - 14)	C_6H_6	(0–200 g/l)	
Fluorinated Systems			
$C_N F_{2N+1} C_2H_4(OC_2H_4)_M OH$	$(C_6F_{13}CH)_2$		
N = 6 - 7	$C_8F_{17}C_2H_5$		10–90°C
M 2, 11 - 14	$C_6F_{13}CH=CH_2$		
$C_8F_{17}C_2H_4N(C_2H_4OH)_2$			

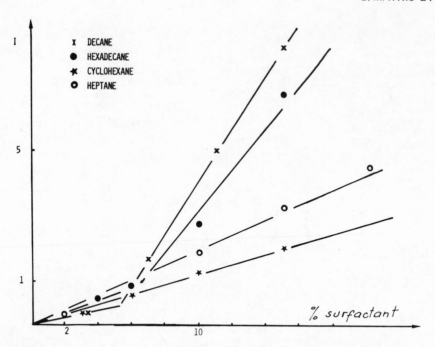

Fig. 1.   Neutron intensity scattered by solutions of $C_{12}(EO)_4$ in four oils, versus the weight concentration of surfactant. Temperature is $20^\circ C$.

tron scattering intensity versus the surfactant concentration. That concentration is about 4-5% in weight, and the aggregation numbers are fairly small. (See Fig. 1.)

For less apolar media or shorter hydrocarbons, for example heptane, cyclohexane, no such a critical concentration can be seen (at $20^\circ C$, using $C_{12}(EO)_4$), but a small progressive aggregation still occurs.

On the other hand, for benzene, chloroform... there is no aggregation at all for the same experimental condition as above.

When that critical concentration exists, the aggregation number n increases if the HLB increases and if the temperature decreases (n is about 10). Thus these variations are opposite to those in the aqueous systems. A hank structure with interdigited hydrophilic chains is very likely.

(b) The C.M.C. of the <u>fluorinated</u> surfactants both in water and in some fluorocarbons have been measured by using the iodine solubili

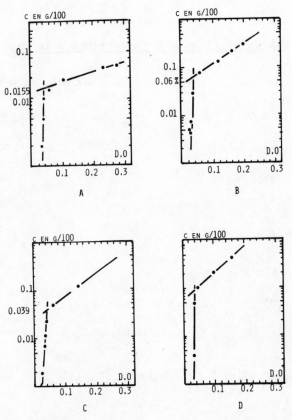

Fig. 2.   A few iodine titration curves of fluorinated surfactants in water.

$$B = C_6F_{13}C_2H_4(OC_2H_4)_{14}OH$$
$$C = C_6F_{13}C_2H_4(OC_2H_4)_{11,5}OH$$
$$D = C_8F_{17}C_2H_4N(C_2H_4OH)_2$$

The curve A is relative to Triton X 100, added for comparison.

zation method[17]. A few titration curves are shown on Fig. 2. A TRITON x 100 titration curve has been added for comparison.

For aqueous solutions, the first two results of Table II demonstrate that, for the same hydrophobic chain, the CMC decreases when the number of oxyethylene decreases. It is the common variation for the hydrogenated surfactants having less than 15 carbon atoms. The classical law log C.M.C. $= A + B.R$, where R is the polyoxyethylene

Table II

C.M.C. of Fluorinated Surfactants in Water

	C.M.C. g/100 ml	C.M.C. Mole/l
$C_6F_{13}CH_2CH_2-(OCH_2CH_2)_{\sim 14}OH$	0.06	$6.12.10^{-4}$
$C_6F_{13}CH_2CH_2-(OCH_2CH_2)_{\sim 11.5}OH$	0.039	$4.48.10^{-4}$
$C_8F_{17}C_2H_4N(C_2H_4OH)_2$	0.009	$1.63.10^{-4}$
$C_{12}H_{25}(OCH_2CH_2)_6OH$		$0.78.10^{-4}$
$C_{12}H_{25}(OCH_2CH_2)_{12}$ at $23^{\circ}C$		$1.4.10^{-4}$

Ln (C.M.C.) = A + B R

$C_{12}H_{25}(OC_2H_4)_nOH$ B = 0.128

$C_6F_{13}C_2H_4(OC_2H_4)_nOH$ B = 0.125

Lipophily $(C_6F_{13}C_2H_4-) \approx$ Lipophily $(C_{12}H_{25}-)$

mole ratio seems also to be suitable. The B value is 0.128 for[18] the hydrogenated surfactants, for the dodecanol derivative. Its value is 0.125 for the fluorinated compound. The influence of the number of oxyethylene groups is then the same[21].

As far as the influence of the hydrophobic chain is concerned, we can see that the second surfactant and the last one have similar values for the C.M.C., the number of the oxyethylene groups being approximately the same. For ionic surfactants, Shinoda[19] has shown that the C.M.C. of fluorinated compounds corresponds to that of a hydrogenated one, but having a hydrophobic chain one point five times longer. Thus it seems to be the same for the nonionic compounds.

The C.M.C. of some fluorinated surfactants in a few fluorocarbons have also been determined (Table III). The diethanolamine has been dissolved in three different solvents. It can be seen that the C.M.C. values increase with Hildebrand's solubility parameters δ [20] of the solvents, which have been evaluated from surface tension data. This expresses the role of the interactions between the solvent and the hydrophobic moieties.

Table III

C.M.C. of Fluorinated Surfactants in Fluorocarbons

		C.M.C. g/100 ml	C.M.C. Mole/l
$C_6F_{13}(CH_2)_3(OC_2H_4)_2OH$	C_6F_6	0.27	$9.33 \ 10^{-3}$
$C_8F_{17}C_2H_4N(C_2H_4OH)_2$	C_6F_6	0.0125	$3.65 \ 10^{-4}$
	$(C_6F_{13}CH)_2$	0.007	$2.25 \ 10^{-4}$
	$C_8F_{17}C_8H_{17}$	0.0034	

For $C_8F_{17}C_2H_4N(C_2H_4OH)_2$:

$$\delta(C_6F_6) > \delta(C_6F_{13}CH)_2 > \delta(C_8F_{17}C_8H_{17})$$

$$C.M.C.(C_6F_6) > C.M.C.(C_6F_{13}CH)_2 > C.M.C. \ (C_8F_{17}C_8H_{17})$$

2) Solubilization Properties

Two types of phase diagrams have been drawn:
- the ternary diagrams for a given temperature,
- and the phase diagram temperature-composition, for a given concentration of surfactant. Where the one, two and three phase regions are drawn (Fig. 3a).

For high contents of water, the upper boundary of the one phase region is the cloud point curve, which indicates the limit of the solubility of the surfactant in water. The lower boundary indicates the maximum oil solubility at a given temperature.

For high contents of oil, the lower boundary is called the haze point curve: it indicates the temperature below which the surfactant is no longer soluble in the oil. The upper boundary is the maximum water solubilization curve. The temperature for which the maximum solubilization of the oil occurs is called the PIT, the phase inversion temperature[1].

According to the surfactant concentration and the salinity, a three phase region of variable extent can exist. A correspondance between the two types of diagrams can be achieved very easily, as schematically shown on Fig. 3a-3b. The two dashed lines correspond to the same temperature and surfactant concentration. The outlook of

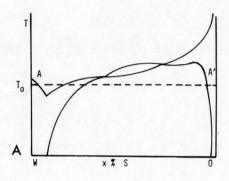

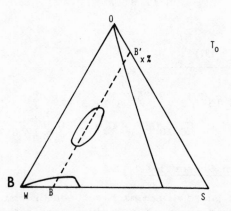

Fig. 3. Schematic representation of the two types of phase diagram.
Lines AA' and BB' correspond to the same temperature and compositions.

that ternary diagram is characteristic of the PIT[22]. When the temperature increases, the ternary phase diagrams take the successive
forms shown on Fig. 4.

According to a given outlook, a linear relation between temperature and HLB can be established (Fig. 5). By using different polyoxyethylene glycol alkyl ethers, the same type of diagram may be
found, but at different temperatures. At least in the neighbourhood
of the PIT, a one unit increase of the HLB is equivalent to a $15^{\circ}C$
decrease of the temperature.

The ternary systems with fluorinated surfactants produce the same
type of temperature-composition diagrams. The solubilization curves
for some fluorocarbons in aqueous solutions, containing 10% of surfactant are shown in Fig. 6.[21]

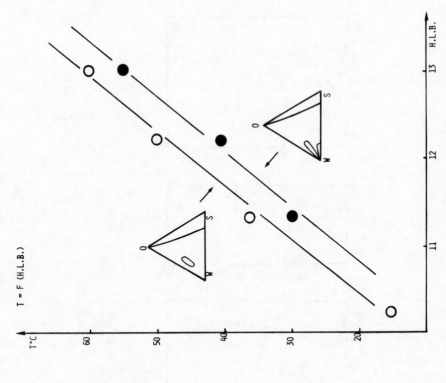

Fig. 5. The linear correspondance HLB-temperature for $C_{12}(EO)_N$, with $N = 4,5,6,7$, in the neighbourhood of the PIT, from the general outlook of the ternary phase diagrams.

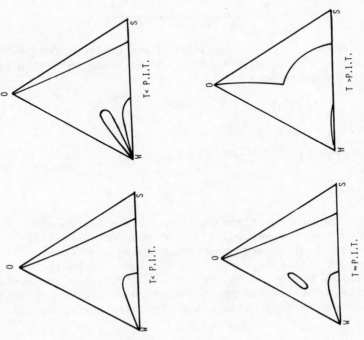

Fig. 4. The successive schematic outlooks of the ternary phase diagrams when the temperature is increasing from below to above the PIT.

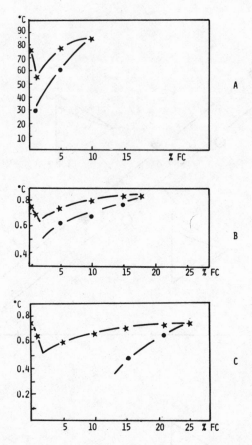

Fig. 6.   Temperature – Composition phase diagrams for the fluorinated surfactant $C_6 F_{13} C_2 H_4 (O C_2 H_4)_{14}$ OH at a concentration of 10%, for different fluorocarbons.

$$A = (C_6 F_{13} CH)_2$$
$$B = \quad C_8 F_{17} C_2 H_5$$
$$C = \quad C_6 F_{13} CH = CH_2$$

When the number of carbon atoms of the fluorocarbon increases, the temperature corresponding to the maximum solubility increases too, and the amount of fluorocarbon solubilized decreases. This is quite analogous to the behaviour of the hydrogenated surfactant. Another similarity is evidenced on Fig. 7: the HLB of the two surfactant systems has been lowered by the addition of a fluorinated alcohol (C curve) or a more lipophilic nonionic surfactant (D curve). And this

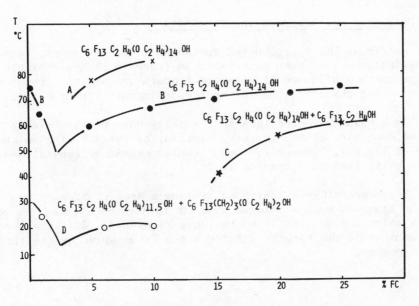

Fig. 7.   Variation of the cloud point with the HLB of the surfactant
system:

A = $(C_6 F_{13} CH)_2$ and aqueous solutions of 10% of

$C_6 F_{13} C_2 H_4 (O C_2 H_4)_{\sim 14} OH$

B = $C_6 F_{13} CH = CH_2$ and aqueous solutions of 10% of

$C_6 F_{13} C_2 H_4 (O C_2 H_4)_{\sim 14} OH$

C = $C_6 F_{13} CH = CH_2$ and aqueous solution of 15% of the
                                         mixture:

$C_6 F_{13} C_2 H_4 (O C_2 H_4)_{\sim 14} OH$ (66%) and:

$C_6 F_{13} C_2 H_4 OH$ (34%)

D = $(C_6 F_{13} CH_2)_2$ and aqueous solution of 5% of the mixture:

$C_6 F_{13} C_2 H_4 (O C_2 H_4)_{\sim 11,5} OH$ (55%) and:

$C_6 F_{13} (C H_2)_3 (O C_2 H_4)_2 OH$ (45%)

decrease of the HLB corresponds to a decrease of the temperature of
the maximum of solubilization.

The comparison of the behaviour of the fluorinated and hydrogenated surfactants suggests that the first ones would be able to form
stable microemulsions at lower temperature, if they were less hydrophilic than those of the present study.

3)   Effect of Salts and of the Temperature

As far as he hydrogenated surfactants are concerned, systematic
investigations have been undertaken in order to obtain reliable information on the influence of both the temperature and the presence of
salts on the phase regions in the pseudo ternary mixtures[23].

As a result, temperature and salinity have a quite similar effect
on the evolution of the ternary diagrams, at least in the neighbourhood of the PIT. [However, these results cannot be generalized for
every salt, like sulfocyanide ...[24]].

The temperature-salinity equivalences are graphically represented
on the Fig. 8: each strip corresponds to a given type of the phase d
grams which may be quantified by the parameter ϕ. ϕ is the percentage
of the area of the ternary diagram which is occupied by the three
phase region.

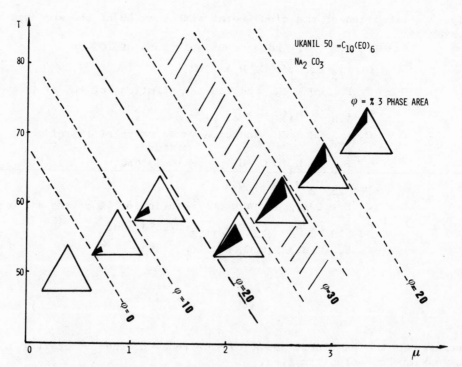

Fig. 8. Temperature-ionic strength (μ) equivalence, from the general
outlook of the ternary phase diagrams.
    Salt   : $Na_2 CO_3$ (C < 150g/1);
    Surfactant : $C_{9-11}(EO)_6$.

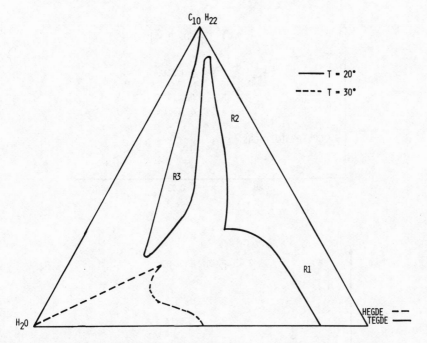

Fig. 9.   Ternary phase diagrams of:

Decane-water-$C_{12}(EO)_4$ at $20^{\circ}C$ (———)
Decane-water-$C_{12}(EO)_6$ at $30^{\circ}C$ (— — —)

As far as the sodium salts are concerned, the chemical nature
of the anion has no great importance. On the other hand, the calcium
salts modify the phase diagrams to a much lesser degree. For sufficiently high values of the temperature and the salinity, the diagrams
may look like WINDSOR'S model.

Although no experiment has been yet fully performed with fluorinated systems, we got some evidence that the influence of salts is
roughly similar.

A full discussion of these results will be published elsewhere.

4)   Structural Investigations

Our work mainly concerns the isotropic phases of the system
decane-tetraethylene glycol dodecyl ether (T.E.G.D.E.)-water at $20^{\circ}C$,
for low content of water. We studied the H.E.G.D.E. for systems with
high content of water. On Fig. 9 is the corresponding phase diagram.

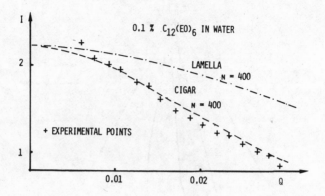

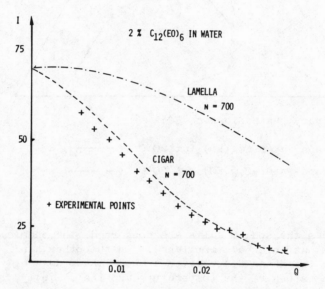

Fig. 10.   Neutron intensity scattered by solutions of O,1% and 2% of $C_{12}(EO)_6$ in water at $30^{\circ}C$.

\+ + + +   experimental curve

——·——   theoretical curve for lamellar model

— — — —   theoretical curve for spherocylindrical model

The techniques which have been used are the light scattering, the
X-ray scattering and the neutron scattering.

First, for the T.E.G.D.E. system, there are three types of structures, respectively for high contents of oil, high contents of surfactant, and in the quasi isolated microemulsions area. Let us note
that the structural problem is highly complex, due to the large interparticular effects and the high sensitivity of the system towards the
temperature and the purity of the surfactant.

a) Let us review very briefly our results with the T.E.G.D.E.

- In the R1 region, we get multilamellar grains, the number of
which is proportional to the water content, above a pseudo C.M.C.[22].
This size and the lamellar thickness have been evaluated. By adding
decane, the hydrophobic parts progressively separate, since the Bragg
distance is increasing from 30 to 60 $\overset{o}{A}$.

- In the R2 region, there are small bilayers, the water being
entrapped along the hydrophilic part of the surfactant. Adding water
causes a rapid increase of the aggregation number, together with a
drastic decrease of the free surfactant concentration.

- In the R3 region, we do have an oil external phase; the water
may form large more or less regular globules.

b) For the hexa-ethylene glycol dodecyl ether (H.E.G.D.E.)
system, in the direct micellar region, the results are rather puzzling.
For a surfactant concentration between 1 and 2%, the aggregates are
probably cylinder-like particles. That can be seen on Fig. 10, from
the curves of the neutron scattering measurements[x]. The crosses are
the experimental results, the lines are the theoretical curves for
sphero cylindrical or lamellar models (orientated at random). D_2O is
used as solvent, for concentrations between 0.1 and 2%. The temperature was 35°C.

At higher surfactant concentration, the aggregation number seems
to decrease, even by taking into account the interparticular effects.

c) If we use homologous fluorinated surfactant of equivalent
HLB, according to Davis' rule in water, we also get particles with an
aggregation number of about 700. Such an aggregation number prevents
any quasi spherical form. On the curves of Fig. 11 are drawn the
theoretical results for the corresponding sphero-cylindrical and lamellar models. Obviously neither of them fits perfectly the experimental curves. But a worm-like shape could be suitable, (the ratio

[x]. The neutron scattering have been performed at Grenoble (F) in the
Laue-Langevin Institute, on D11 and D17 apparatus.

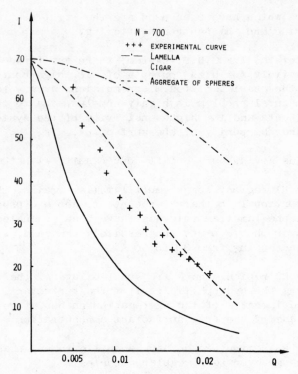

Fig. 11. Neutron intensity scattered by a solution of 0,1% of fluorinated surfactant.

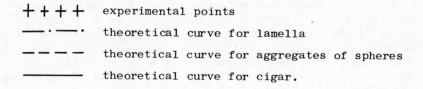

+ + + +   experimental points

— · — ·   theoretical curve for lamella

— — — —   theoretical curve for aggregates of spheres

—————   theoretical curve for cigar.

length to diameter should be about 40) if its radius of gyration is about one third of the radius of gyration of the straight sphero-cylindrical particle. There is another possible model: that of an extended aggregate of about a few tens of small spheres. Indeed the theoretical curve of the scattering intensity for a random chain of 70 spheres is shown on Fig. 11[25]. That number of spheres is coherent with the aggregation number (700), and the radius of gyration (100 Å) corresponds to a distance between the centers of the spheres of about 30 Å. In fact, some polydispersity should occur (for example, the number of spheres could be between 40 and 100) for a better fitting of the experimental curve. We cannot now choose between the two possibilities. In short, it appears from our few

structural studies that the two types of nonionic surfactants have
also very similar morphological properties.

REFERENCES

1. K Shinoda, Solvent properties of surfactant solutions. Ed.
    M. Dekker (1967).
2. K. Shinoda and H. Kuneida, J. Colloid Interface Sci., 42, 381
    (1973).
3. K. Shinoda and S. Friberg, Adv. in Colloid and Interface Sci.,
    4, 281 (1975).
4. S. Friberg and I. Lapczynska, Prog. Colloid Polymer Sci., 56, 16
    (1975).
5. S. Friberg, I. Lapczynska and G. Gillberg, J. Colloid Interface
    Sci., 56, 19 (1976).
6. R. R. Balmbra, J. S. Clunie, J. M. Corkill and J. F. Goodman
    Trans. Faraday Soc. 58, 1661 (1962).
7. R. R. Balmbra, J. S. Clunie, J. M. Corkill and J. F. Goodman
    ibid, 60, 979 (1964).
8. P. H. Elworthy and C. B. Macfarlane, J. Chem. Soc., 907 (1963).
9. J. M. Corkill and T. Walker, J. Colloid Interface Sci., 39, 621
    (1972).
10. R. H. Ottewill, C. C. Storer and T. Walker, Trans. Faraday Soc.,
    63, 2796 (1967).
11. J. M. Corkill, J. F. Goodman and J. Wyer, ibid, 65, 9, (1969).
12. J. S. Clunie, J. F. Goodman, P. C. Symons, ibid, 65, 287 (1969).
13. For a review of the modern techniques see:
    - B. Lindman and H. Wennerstrom, Physics Reports, 52, 1 (1979).
    - G. J. T. Tiddy, Physics Reports, 57, 1, (1980).
14. G. Mathis, J. C. Boubel, J. J. Delpuech, J. C. Ravey and M. Buzier
    Proceedings of the Second International Congress on NMR in
    Colloid and Interface Science, ed. Reidel Pub. Comp. p.597 (1980).
15. M. J. Schick, Nonionic surfactants, Ed. M. Dekker (1966).
16. For a review see: H. F. Eicke, in "Topics in current chemistry-
    micelles", Ed. Springer Verlag, 87 (1979), and A. S. Kertes in
    "Micellization, solubilization and microemulsions", Vol. 1, Ed.
    K. Mittal, Plenum Press (1977).
17. S. Ross and J. P. Olivier, J. Phys. Chem. 63, 1671 (1959).
18. H. Lange, Proc. 3 Intern. Congr. Surface Activity, Köln, 1,
    279 (1960).
19.a K. Shinoda, M. Hato and T. Hayashi, J. Phys. Chem., 76, 909,
    (1972).
19.b H. Kuneida and S. Shinoda, J. Phys. Chem., 80, 2468 (1976).
20. J. H. Hildebrand and R. L. Scott, "The solubility of non electro-
    lytes", 3rd Ed. Dover Publ. Inc., N.Y. (1964).
21. G. Mathis, Thèse Docteur Ingénieur Nancy (1978).
22. S. Friberg, I. Buraczewska, J. C. Ravey, in "Micellization,
    solubilization and microemulsions", Vol.2, Ed. K. Mittal, Plenum
    Press (1977).
23. M. Buzier, Thèse spécialité, Nancy (1978).

24. K. Shinoda, private communication.
25. J. C. Ravey, J. Colloid Interface Sci., 50, 545 (1975).

DISCUSSION

Dr. P. R. Rowland: You mentioned effects measured in D_2O. Did they differ from those for H_2O? If so, is there a model for this?

Dr. J. C. Ravey: They did not differ.

DIELECTRIC STUDIES OF A NONIONIC SURFACTANT-ALKANE-WATER SYSTEM AT LOW WATER CONTENT

M. H. Boyle[+], M. P. McDonald[++], P. Rossi[++] and R. M. Wood[+]

[+] Department of Applied Physics
[++] Department of Chemistry

Sheffield City Polytechnic

INTRODUCTION

It has been shown by Friberg[1] that the heptane-water-tetraoxy-ethylene glycol dodecyl ether ($C_{12}E_4$) system forms clear single phases over appreciable ranges of composition and temperature. Within such a clear phase, the micelles may be normal (i.e. oil in water) or reversed (i.e. water in oil) and in some instances a transformation occurs from the former to the latter with change in temperature or composition without departure from the single phase region.

The dielectric properties of these systems have received little attention. Clausse et al[2] studied benzene in water with the nonionic surfactants Tween 20 and Span 20 as emulsifiers. Dielectric dispersion was not observed and the dielectric behaviour was attributed to interfacial polarisation. Experimental data was in accordance with predictions obtained with the Hanai equation[3] for an oil in water emulsion. Peyrelasse et al[4] observed pronounced dispersion in water in undecane microemulsions with blends of polyexyethylene octyl phenyl ethers. Again, large dispersion was observed by Peyrelasse et al[5] in water in hexadecane microemulsions. This dispersion was attributed to interfacial polarisation and it was proposed that reversed micelles were present, the surfactant head groups in the surface of which made an admittance contribution.

In contrast, in the case of ionic surfactants with benzene and water, Eicke and Shepherd[6] favoured an interpretation based on the orientation of micelles in the applied electric field with changes being attributed to micellar aggregation. Previous dielectric work performed in this laboratory on the clear single phases in approxima-

103

tely 2:3 w/w alkane-water mixtures containing up to 20% $C_{12}E_4$ has
shown different behaviours as the alkane chain length increased from
seven to sixteen carbon atoms. In all instances did the phases appear
to be microemulsions and the differences in behaviour are ascribed to
changes in the shape of the dispersed phase and to partial or total
inversion from normal to reverse micelles. These results are consistent with the observations and conclusions of Bostock et al[7] for the
same regions of the same systems where the investigation technique was
electrical conductance measurement.

The work now reported relates to mixtures in the low water content region of the diagram for the system $C_{12}E_4$-water-heptane and was
carried out to ascertain to what extent the behaviour observed in the
$C_{12}E_4$-water binary and that in the ternary at high water content is
mirrored in the clear phase containing little water.

EXPERIMENTAL

Tetraoxyethylene glycol dodecyl ether ($C_{12}E_4$) was obtained from
Nikkol Chemicals, Japan; the water was double distilled and the heptane was I P normal grade (BDH). Measurements were made at 2 MHz
using a WTW Dipolmeter and cells MFL 2 and DFL 2, both of which had
been calibrated using standard liquids. Temperature was controlled to
$\pm$ 0.2°C and measured permittivities carry a precision of $\pm$ 0.01.
Required mixtures of the component liquids were prepared using a precision balance giving a maximum uncertainty in the mass fraction of
0.002.

RESULTS AND DISCUSSION

Figure 1 shows three isothermal sections of the $C_{12}E_4$-C_7H_{16}-H_2O
phase diagram. The isotropic clear liquid regions are those contained
within the dashed lines or between a dashed line and the diagram bound
ary. At 1°C there is a clear region on the left of the diagram which
decreases in size at higher temperatures and then disappears completely at 8°C. By 13°C another clear region has appeared rather nearer
the heptane corner. Between 13°C and 39°C the right hand region con-
tinues to expand, makes contact with the left hand region and then the
combined regions withdraw towards the heptane-surfactant boundary,
leaving a sharp peninsula as shown in this section. At the lower temperatures, there is also a very small region of isotropic solution
close to the water corner. As will be seen later, most of the dielectric data was obtained within the temperature range 10°C to 50°C
although three compositions were examined close to 0°C. As a reference point the phase inversion temperature (PIT) of a mixture of equal
volumes of heptane and an aqueous solution of 0.005M KCl containing
2% $C_{12}E_4$ was found conductimetrically to be 10.3°C. (The presence of
0.005M KCl has been found to have no measureable effect on the phase
behaviour of the $C_{12}E_4$-H_2O system.).

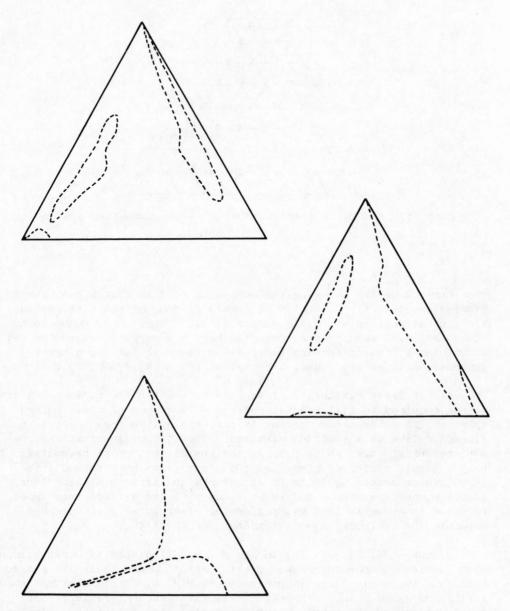

Figure 1.   Section of phase diagram of tetraoxyethylene glycol dodecyl
ether–heptane–water system at 1°C, 13°C and 39°C.   Clear isotropic
single phase regions identified by the letter L.

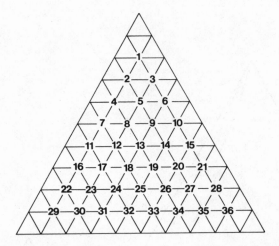

Figure 2: Triangular diagram showing sample numbering system.

Our scheme for studying the behaviour of this system has been to
examine samples at regular 10% intervals of composition with, in addition, occasional intermediate compositions. Samples are numbered as
shown in Fig. 2 and the work reported here was carried out on the set
containing 10% water forming the rows on the right of the diagram
(exceptionally sample number 3 contained 16% $C_{12}E_4$/74% C_7H_{16}).

All of these mixtures contain less water than the minimum 26% by
volume required to fill the interstices of a system of close packed
spheres. Thus the water content is insufficient to form the sole continuous medium in any of the mixtures. It will be seen that the present set of mixtures which display the common feature of presenting
only a single region of clear isotropic phase can be arranged into
three groups according to their structures and structural behaviour.
Sample number 7 was reported on previously[8] and differs from those
referred to above in that two regions of clear phase were observed
separated by a cloudy phase extending over about 4°C.

Mixtures 36, 28, 21, 15, 10 and 6 were all stable as clear single
phases over a temperature range of at least 30°C and their dielectric
behaviour over this range is presented in Fig. 3. These mixtures show
similar rates of change of permittivity with temperature (although
the curvature of the graphs change slightly), indicating that similar
processes are probably occurring in all of them. For these mixtures,
the water is always ≤ 25% by weight of the water + surfactant content,
for which composition range the binary surfactant-water system also
shows appreciable temperature ranges of simgle phase behaviour; Fig. 4
displays this. NMR self-diffusion measurements at temperatures

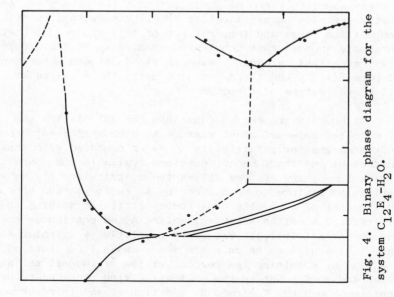

Fig. 4. Binary phase diagram for the system $C_{12}E_4$-H_2O.

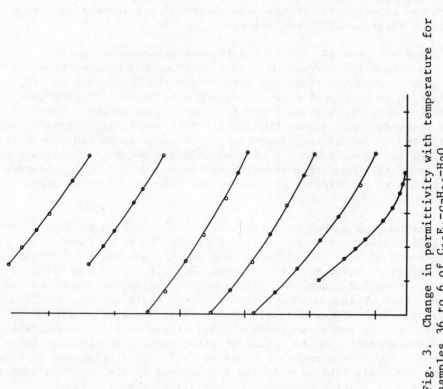

Fig. 3. Change in permittivity with temperature for samples 36 to 6 of $C_{12}E_4$-C_7H_{16}-H_2O.

between about 50°C and 65°C suggest that the binary surfactant-water system contains normal micelles at all concentrations within the above composition range and temperatures of this order[7]. Dielectric measurements support this conclusion at high surfactant contents (> 70% w/w), excellent agreement being obtained between experimental values of permittivity and those computed using the Hanai equation for an oil in water type of structure[8].

Although there are no equations for calculating the permittivity of an oil-water-surfactant mixture at high surfactant content, the very much greater permittivity of water compared with those of oil and surfactant and the form of equations available for computing permittivities for binary systems allows the distribution of the water in a particular mixture to be deduced by an approximation approach (water in the core of a micelle contributes little or nothing to the permittivity of a micellar solution; water in the continuous medium dominates the permittivity). Values of permittivity calculated (i) using the Hanai equations on only the water and oil contents of the mixtures and (ii) by combining the permittivities of the oil and surfactant or water and surfactant as though ideal mixing occurred to produce the continuous medium, followed by addition of the third component as the dispersed phase in the Hanai equations may be compared in Table 1 with the experimental values at each end of the temperature range over which a clear solution was obtained.

For mixtures 36, 28, 21 and 15, the experimental permittivities are less than the corresponding O/W+S values but greater than the W/O +S ones. Consistent with the results for the binary system, this situation is interpreted as indicating a structure in which oil-cored micelles exist in a water-surfactant continuous medium. The fact that the water does not appear to make its full permittivity contibution to the value of the mixture ($\varepsilon_{exp} < \varepsilon_{O/W+S}$) is taken to indicate restriction of the water molecules by their binding to the EO_4 chains. For the range of composition involved in these four mixtures, the number of bound water molecules per surfactant molecule increases from about 2.5 to 4.

Although a number of workers have discussed the binding of water to polyethylene oxide chains, there appears to be no fixed value for the amount of water bound to an EO group and according to Schott[9], the quantity varies with surfactant. Recently Kumar and Balasubramanian[10] using a number of different measuring techniques on the same system, Triton X-100, hexanol, water, cyclohexanol, have found that in hydrocarbon-rich mixtures the first added water goes to hydrate the polyethylene oxide chains; at higher water contents the evidence suggests the formation of water pools. The results indicate that the EO_{10} chain probably takes up to 16 water molecules of hydration, the equivalent of which in the present system is the accommodation of 5 or 6 water molecules of hydration by an EO_4 chain.

In contrast with the mixtures referred to above, those numbered

Table 1

Comparison of Calculated and Experimental Permittivity Values

Mixture Number	Temp °C	εs	Calculated Permittivity			
			O/W	W/O	O/(W+S)	W/(O+S)
36	15.2	9.63	23.79	9.40	12.37	7.35
	47.6	8.36	19.69	8.75	10.10	6.65
28	15.2	8.39	14.06	4.96	11.47	6.62
	47.9	7.20	11.64	4.64	9.43	5.96
21	1.0	7.48	9.98	3.67	10.41	6.12
	48.1	5.94	7.90	3.41	8.19	5.19
15	1.1	6.52	9.43	3.18	9.15	5.28
	48.3	4.92	6.30	2.96	7.52	4.64
10	0.9	5.86	6.92	2.96	8.30	4.65
	48.0	3.98	5.55	2.76	6.72	4.14
6	10.8	4.86	5.48	2.66	7.03	3.93
	42.9	3.52	5.00	2.59	6.07	3.65
3	17.8	3.90	5.02	2.56	4.52	3.24
	31.3	2.99	4.52	2.45	4.38	3.16
1	16.7	3.26	4.68	2.48		
	23.0	2.74	4.61	2.47		
2	14.3	4.65	8.50	3.38		
	17.1	3.63	8.42	3.38		
4	12.0	7.64	13.63	4.79		
	15.4	4.63	13.43	4.76		
5	17.9	5.26	9.40	3.63		
	23.8	3.86	9.14	3.61		
7	5.7	21.98	20.90	7.40		
	7.3	20.39	20.78	7.40		
	12.0	9.22	20.37	7.40		
	13.4	6.43	20.24	7.36		

one to five have low surfactant contents and hence their clear regions
might be expected to have a microemulsion structure. Their dielectric
behaviours are presented in Fig. 5 where it can be seen that numbers
two, four and five show a high rate of change of permittivity with
temperature while the other two mixtures have a much smaller rate of
change. In all five instances, the temperature range over which the
clear region forms and which is close to the PIT is considerably smaller than that of the previous considered set. Mixtures 1, 2, 4 and 5
have upper temperature limit experimental permittivities which agree
well with the calculated ones for a W/O structure when the mixtures are
treated as binaries of oil and water and the Hanai equation is applied.
All of the set, one to five (and 6) contain greater than 60% by volume
of heptane. The absence of a separate low temperature clear liquid
region as appears in mixture number 7 suggests that it is not possible
to solubilise such large quantities of heptane even as a microemulsion
because of the relatively small amounts of water present[8]. Allowing
for the minimum hydration of $C_{12}E_4$ suggested above and assuming all
hydrated surfactant molecules occupy interfacial regions, there will
be little free water left to form a continuous medium.

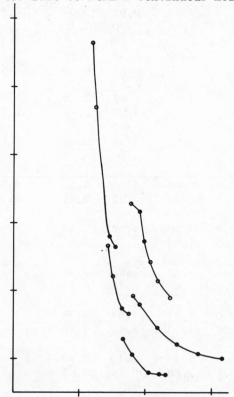

Fig. 5. Change in permittivity with temperature for samples 1 to 5
of $C_{12}E_4-C_7H_{16}-H_2O$.

Mixtures 1 and 3 have been observed to form a single lamellar liquid crystal (l.c.) phase at temperatures lower than those of the present clear phases. Also, the water/surfactant ratios of all mixtures one to five (and 6) lie in the range in which lamellar l.c. phase is stable in the binary system (Fig. 3). Accordingly, it is suggested that in mixtures, 1, 2, 4 and 5 the l.c. phase has become an arrangement of large lamellar aggregates at the lower temperature end of the clear phase range which, on increase of temperature, change to inverted micelles.

At the high surfactant end of the set of mixtures, all of the water was claimed earlier in this presentation to be bound to the polyethylene oxide chains while at the composition of mixture 1, the above evidence is that "pools" of water are involved. Thus at some composition between these, the first unbound or free water must appear. Mixtures 6 and 3 have similar behaviour in the lower temperature region of their clear ranges in that they both exhibit streaming birefringence and their dielectric permittivities as given in Table 1 fit an O/W+S structure in which the water is bound. At the higher temperature end of the range, their experimental permittivities show good agreement with values calculated for a W/O+S structure, but are slightly less than these values in each instance.

It is proposed that the bound water molecules of the present high surfactant content mixtures become "freer" as the hydrogen bonding decreases on increasing the mixture temperature until the water is unable to be accommodated in molecular form. When the hydrogen bonding breaks down and the entropy of mixing is insufficient, the water becomes encapsulated. Such a process of inversion would not be expected to occur while the composition of a mixture is such that all of the water can be bound to EO_4 chains throughout the temperature range of the clear phase. Calculation shows that at the composition of mixture 10 there are five water molecules for each $C_{12}E_4$ molecule which fits well with the previously referred to maximum hydration values of five to six deduced from the work of Kumar and Balasubramanian[10] and so it is around this composition that inversion to a W/O type structure might be expected to be observed. As Table 1 shows, the experimental permittivity of mixture 10 at the low temperature end of the range is greater than the calculated values for a W/O+S structure but less than that for the O/W+S. As with the higher surfactant content mixtures, this is taken to indicate oil cored micelles in a water plus surfactant continuous medium where the water is bound. At the higher temperature end of the range of clear phase, this mixture is the one with the lowest water to surfactant ratio to display a permittivity appropriate to a W/O+S structure. Thus it is concluded that inversion does occur in this mixture and that it is in accordance with the controlling mechanism suggested above.

CONCLUSIONS

As the surfactant content of the mixtures $(C_{12}E_4-C_7H_{16}-H_2O)$ decreases from 80% to 10% at constant 10% water, there is a progressive change in structure and structural behaviour of the clear isotropic single phase. At high surfactant contents the structure is O/W+S with the water bound to the EO_4 chains throughout the temperature range of existence. At intermediate and low surfactant contents inversion occurs within the clear single phase region, the mechanism of inversion being controlled by a combination of decreasing hydrogen bonding and increasing entropy of mixing with an insufficiency of the latter as a critical requirement. The low water content tends to result in an O/W+S structure with the water bound at low temperatures of the range becoming W/O+S at higher temperatures. Higher water content at low surfactant compositions encourages formation of a lamellar or very oblate micelle structure at lower temperatures in the clear phase range.

REFERENCES

1. S. Friberg, I. Lapczynska, Progr. Colloid and Polymer Sci. 56, 16, (1975).
2. M. Clausse, P. Sherman, R. J. Sheppard, J. Colloid Interface Sci. 56, 123 (1976).
3. T. Hanai, "Emulsion Science" (P. Sherman, Ed) Academic Press, London/New York 1968 p.353.
4. J. Peyrelasse, C. Boned, P. Xans, M. Clausse, C. R. Acad. Sci. Paris B 284, 235 (1977).
5. J. Peyrelasse, V. E. R. McClean, C. Boned, R. J. Sheppard, M. Clausse, J. Phys. D. Appl. Phys. 11, L117 (1978).
6. H. F. Eicke, J. C. W. Shepherd, Helv. Chem. Acta. 57, 1951 (1974).
7. T. A. Bostock, M. P. McDonald, G. J. T. Tiddy, L. Waring, SCI Chemical Society Symposium on Surface Active Agents, Nottingham 1979.
8. T. A. Bostock, M. H. Boyle, M. P. McDonald, R. M. Wood. J. Colloid Interface Sci. 73 368 (1980).
9. H. Schott, J. Colloid Interface Sci. 24, 193 (1980).
10. C. Kumar, D. Balasubramanian, J. Colloid Interface Sci., 74, 64, (1980).

DISCUSSION

Dr I. D. Robb: Does the area of the phase diagram where the water is not "bulk water" increase in size with decreasing temperature and does the dielectric data correspond to diffuse physical boundaries between water and surfactant?

Dr R. M. Wood: In reply to your first question, I interpret your description "not bulk water" as referring to the set of samples containing 10% water. The area on the phase diagram in which this set of samples lies and which has been identified as defining a clear single phase changes in two ways with increase in temperature.

(i) The area existing at 0°C expands in the direction of greater surfactant content until at about 17°C there is clear single phase at all oil-surfactant ratios and 10% water; above this temperature the area decreases in size.

(ii) At each oil-surfactant ratio the quantity of water accomodated in the clear phase increases up to about 25°C above which it decreases.

These behaviours may both be interpreted in terms of the requirement of the oil for an increase in one or other of the additional constituents for its containment on increasing its temperature, possibly until a situation favourable to inversion is set up.

Table 1 shows that the assumption of distinct normal and reversed micellar structures leads to calculated dielectric permittivities which are of clearly different sizes and which change significantly with composition and temperature. Less sharply defined structures would be expected to produce the smaller changes in permittivity which can be observed in the experimental results and so the boundaries between surfactant and water in these mixtures might be described as diffuse or even non-existent.

Dr I. D. Robb: Do you go from systems having water in pools to just water of hydration without crossing a phase boundary?

Dr R. M. Wood: As far as the experimental data has been analysed at present, a similar structure forms at similar temperatures in mixtures having not very dissimilar compositions. However, an increase in temperature brings about inversion in some mixtures and not in others, from which it may be deduced that either a change in temperature or a change in both composition and temperature is necessary for passing from a structure containing "pools" of water to one in which there is water of hydration alone. Such a change is not normally accorded the distinction of a conventional phase boundary.

Prof H. F. Eicke: Partial or total phase inversion should be accompanied by a remarkable change in the complex permittivity (= conductivity), since the system is expected to pass a so-called bicontinuous state proceeding from a W/O to a O/W microemulsion. Could the authors comment?

Dr R. M. Wood: In our as yet unpublished study of inversion in aqueous systems of $C_{12}E_4$ with heptane and with decane at microemulsion compositions we have observed large decreases in permittivity when O/W structures change to W/O. The magnitudes of the changes contrast with those of the present work, even in the case of sample number 4 which shows the largest effect of temperature. The large change in permittivity is associated with a high water content (~ 50% W/W) which can provide a water-continuous medium for the O/W structure and so which would appear to make redundant any requirement for an intermediate bicontinuous structure. In the present set of results, mixtures which invert undergo only a small permittivity change on changing the temperature because of their limited water content and its small dielectric contribution. The presence of dissolved ions in a mixture serves to reduce the water contribution, both to the overall permittivity of a mixture and to the change occurring on inversion.

ON THE STRUCTURE AND DYNAMICS OF MICROEMULSIONS

SELF-DIFFUSION STUDIES

B. Lindman[a], N. Kamenka[b], B. Brun[b] and P. G. Nilsson[a]

[a]Physical Chemistry 1, Chemical Center
Lund University, S-220 07 Lund, Sweden

[b]Laboratoire des Interactions Moléculaires
Faculté des Sciences, USTL, Montpellier, France

INTRODUCTION

The thermodynamic stability of microemulsions being well
established[1-3] it is natural to consider structural and molecular
properties of microemulsions in relation to other stable phases which
form in surfactant systems[4-6]. There is unfortunately quite a bit
of confusion about the term microemulsions, being used by some
authors even for typical micelles of the normal or reversed type.
Here our interest will focus on fluid isotropic phases which contain
simultaneously high amounts of water and oil, the latter in a broad
sense, i.e. a compound with very low aqueous solubility like a hydrocarbon or a long-chain alcohol. As one moves in the phase diagram
from very high to very low water contents one must for a strongly
associating system encounter some type of transition from normal to
reversed type aggregates. This article reports on an attempt to use
self-diffusion studies to contribute to our understanding of the
structure and dynamics of such "transition" aggregates. Solutions of
this type are found in "classical" microemulsions formed in four-
component systems ionic surfactant - cosurfactant (normally a short-
chain alcohol) - hydrocarbon-water[7]. However, it is logical to
consider in parallel also other systems with fluid isotropic phases
containing at the same time high concentrations of water and hydrocarbon. A typical example is Shinoda's "surfactant phase" found in
three-component systems nonionic surfactant-hydrocarbon-water[8].
For certain three-component ionic amphiphile systems one also
encounters microemulsion type behaviour. This may occur for surfactant systems where the third component is more strongly hydrophilic,
like the hexadecyltrimethylammonium bromide-butanol-water (9) and
sodium octanoate-octanoic acid-water[10] systems, or when the associa-

115

tion in aqueous solutions is not strongly cooperative and does not lead to typical micelles, like the sodium cholate-decanol-water system(11). In discussing microemulsion systems it is important to recognise that in "typical" three-component surfactant systems one obtains under corresponding conditions a liquid crystalline phase, most frequently a lamellar one.

THE SELF-DIFFUSION METHOD AS A STRUCTURAL TOOL

Within a micelle, molecular motion is almost as rapid as in a liquid hydrocarbon and likewise in a reversed micelle water molecules and counterions are very mobile(12,13). In a lamellar liquid crystal the motion of all components appears to be very rapid in the direction of the lamella while in the perpendicular direction translation diffusion is slow(14). In fact, it appears to be a general feature of amphiphilic systems that all components move freely within a domain(6,13). It is characteristic of amphiphilic systems that there is typically a rather sharp spatial separation between hydrophilic and hydrophobic regions. In such a situation the passage of a molecule or ion between different regions is an improbable event and thus occurs slowly. This has the consequence that in studies of self-diffusion over macroscopic distances, diffusion can be rapid or slow depending exclusively on the geometrical properties of the inner structure of the phase. If a phase is water- but not oil-continuous one expects diffusion of hydrophilic components to be rapid and of hydrophobic components to be slow. For a case with oil- but not water-continuous structure the converse situation should apply. A bicontinuous phase should give rapid diffusion of all components.

These principles we applied some years ago in studies of the structure of cubic liquid crystals(15). Here essentially two types of structure (or a combination of these) had been proposed(16-20). In one, small closed aggregates of the amphiphile are close-packed in a water-continuum or in the reverse situation small "droplets" of water are close-packed in an amphiphile continuum. In the other, there is a network of one of the components extending over macroscopic distances in the other. The two-component system dodecyltrimethylammonium chloride-water was taken as suitable to test structural models since it has two different cubic liquid crystals appearing at different compositions (Fig. 1). In the water-rich one, amphiphile diffusion is very slow (ca. 5.10^{-13} m^2/s), demonstrating the presence of closed amphiphile aggregates between which the amphiphile ions exchange very slowly. In the water-poor one, amphiphile diffusion is much more rapid (ca. 5.10^{-12} m^2/s) giving evidence that the phase is amphiphile-continuous in agreement with a structural model put forth by Luzzati(16,17). It was argued previously and has also been argued more recently(21-24) that this so-called viscous isotropic phase contains close-packed amphiphile globules in a water-continuum but this is ruled out by the self-diffusion data(15,25). The most important argument for small closed aggregates was the appearance of narrow

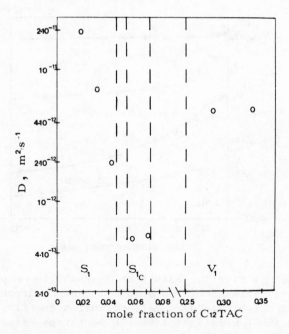

Fig. 1. The amphiphile self-diffusion coefficient in the dodecyl-trimethylammonium chloride (C_{12}TAC)-water system is an order of magnitude larger in the V_1 cubic phase than in the S_{1C} cubic phase, for which it corresponds to the extrapolated values of micellar solutions (S_1). (From Ref. 15).

signals in proton NMR spectra. However, this is not a valid argument since any isotropic phase because of the rapid lateral diffusion should give narrow lines[25].

An important property of these cubic phases is their extremely high viscosity which is consistent with a well-ordered structure where the aggregates themselves are rather rigid and strongly hindered in their motion; the X-ray diffraction pattern observed, of course, directly demonstrates the ordered structure. With refinements of the diffusion technique it has recently been possible to distinguish between different possible bicontinuous structures using information on the lateral diffusion in an oriented lamellar phase[26].

SELF-DIFFUSION IN NORMAL AND REVERSED MICELLAR SOLUTIONS

The self-diffusion coefficients of amphiphile ion (D_A), counterion (D_M), coion (D_X) (of added electrolyte), water (D_W) and solubilizate (D_S) have been studied for a number of ionic surfactant-water systems with similar results for all cases. In Fig. 2 we give the concentration dependence of the self-diffusion coefficients of water, sodium,

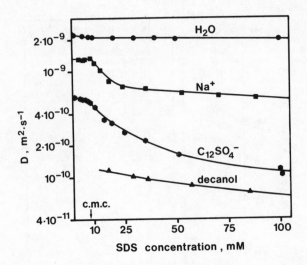

Fig. 2. For normal micellar solutions hydrophilic components (water and counterions) diffuse much more rapidly than hydrophobic ones (surfactant and solubilizate). Self-diffusion coefficients for sodium dodecylsulfate (SDS) solutions taken in part from Refs. 27-29.

dodecyl-sulfate and decanol (added small amounts of decanol) for sodium dodecyl-sulfate solutions. The detailed concentration dependence gives information on the composition of the aggregates formed (counterion binding, hydration etc.) but this aspect will not be discussed here. Here we note only that the high D_W values and the low D_S values demonstrate that in the concentration range studied these solutions are water continuous and oil discontinuous. Most of the dodecylsulfate ions become micellized at higher concentration and therefore D_A approaches D_S. The counterions are dissociated to a considerable degree even at high concentrations and therefore D_M remains large.

Reversed micellar solutions have as yet been investigated to a much smaller extent but the data in Fig. 3 will probably show to be typical. Over a wide concentration range in the L_2 phase of the system sodium octanoate-decanol-water it can be seen that D_A and D_S both are somewhat below 10^{-10} m^2s^{-1} over a wide concentration range while D_M lies in the range 1-$1.5.10^{-11}$ m^2s^{-1}. D_W is higher but also considerably below D_A and D_S. (To correct, very roughly, from mere size effects the data are in Fig. 3 given relative to "standard states" which are the pure liquid for water and decanol or the ions at infinite dilutions in water). From this we may draw the conclusion that below 90% of decanol, the solutions are with good approximation oil-continuous but water-discontinuous. This agrees with the current view of

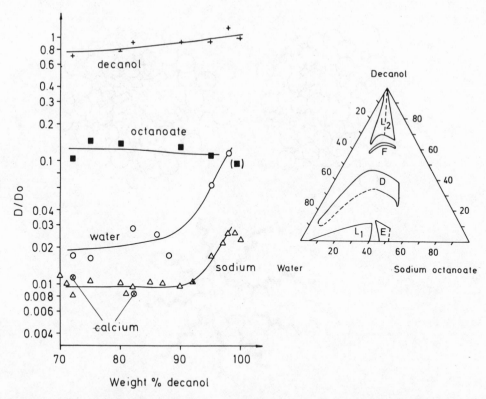

Fig. 3. For reversed micellar solutions hydrophilic components'
(water and counterions) self-diffusion is strongly retarded while
hydrophobic species (surfactant and solubilizate) diffuse considerably
more rapidly. Relative self-diffusion coefficients, i.e. observed
self-diffusion coefficients divided by the values of pure liquids or
infinitely dilute aqueous ions, for the system sodium octonoate-
decanol-water. Sample compositions indicated by the dashed line in
the insert phase diagram (from Ekwall[4] after modification). Calcium
ion diffusion data were obtained on small amounts of added calcium
chloride. (Ref. 30.).

reversed micellar solutions as solutions with separated water globules
containing the counterions in a continuum of decanol containing part
of the surfactant ions, the rest of the surfactant ions and some decanol being at the surface of the water globules.

These observations (which remain to be generalized) indicate that
for a typical three-component system of a surfactant, a predominantly
hydrophobic "solubilizate" and water the two fluid isotropic phases
occurring in the phase diagram contain small globules of water or

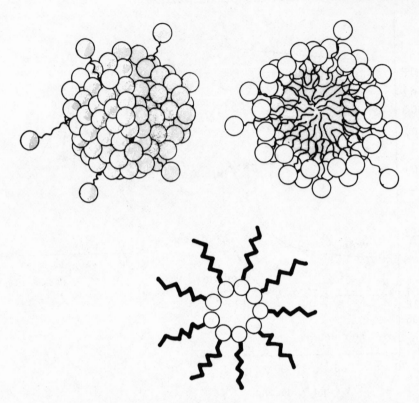

Fig. 4. Typical normal (top) or reversed surfactant micelles have a relatively well-defined hard interface.

amphiphile + solubilizate dispersed in the other component. The globules have a relatively well-defined or "hard" interface (Fig. 4). This has also been amply demonstrated from X-ray diffraction and NMR studies to apply for the liquid crystalline phases (lamellar, hexagonal and cubic) in the same systems[4,16,25,31].

SELF-DIFFUSION IN AN IONIC SURFACTANT MICROEMULSION SYSTEM

Several physico-chemical methods are presently applied to microemulsion systems of the type ionic surfactant-short-chain alcohol-hydrocarbon-water by different laboratories. There are slight differences between the different systems studied but these should be relatively insignificant in particular as regards solution structure. Ourselves we have chosen to study the system sodium octylbenzenesulfonate-pentanol-decane-water-sodium chloride. As may be inferred from Fig. 5 both water, decane and sodium ions have quite high self-diffu-

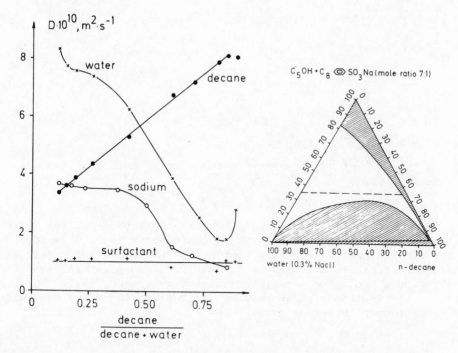

Fig. 5. For an ionic microemulsion system (sodium octyl benzene-sulfonate-pentanol-decane-water-sodium chloride), both hydrophilic and hydrophobic components diffuse quite rapidly over wide concentration ranges. Sample compositions indicated by the dashed line in the schematic phase diagram. (From Ref. 32.).

sion coefficients over an extensive concentration range of the isotropic "microemulsion" phase. In particular they rule out the presence of hard surface closed water or oil globules at typical microemulsion compositions. It is only at quite high water concentrations that D_S approaches D_A and at quite high decane concentrations that D_M approaches D_A. As argued above one expects for typical normal micelles D_S to fall well below D_A and for typical reversed micelles D_M to be much smaller than D_A.

SELF-DIFFUSION IN A NONIONIC SURFACTANT MICROEMULSION SYSTEM

At a particular temperature in a phase diagram of a nonionic surfactant-hydrocarbon-water system there may be three separate regions with fluid isotropic phases (Fig. 6). (In a three-dimensional temperature-composition diagram these are connected). One of these extends from the water corner, one from the hydrocarbon-surfactant base and one, the "surfactant phase", has high concentrations of all three components.

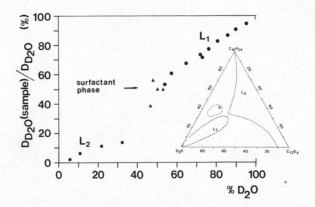

Fig. 6. Water self-diffusion in the surfactant phase of the system
tetraethyleneglycoldodecylether-hexadecane-water is very rapid and
corresponds approximately to a simple obstruction effect. Self-diffusion coefficients measured by ^{2}H NMR (D_2O) and given relative to
that of pure D_2O. The insert indicates very schematically the location of the isotropic phase regions; in reality the phase extensions
are very temperature-sensitive.

The surfactant phase, as well as the extended regions of the other
phases, has a very limited temperature existence range. In Fig. 6
we present the water self-diffusion data for one three-component
system, tetraethylene-glycoldodecylether-hexadecane-water (D_2O). The
results for the different phases have been obtained at slightly different temperatures (and hydrocarbon-to-surfactant ratios), but are in
the figure normalized by dividing with the self-diffusion coefficient
of pure water at the appropriate temperature. It can be seen that the
water molecules diffuse quite rapidly in the surfactant phase and that
there is certainly no discontinuity as one passes from the water-rich
phase (L_1) to the surfactant phase. Also for the hydrocarbon and the
surfactant, diffusion in the surfactant phase is very rapid. Transport studies by Tiddy and co-workers[33] have also demonstrated rapid
translational motion of different species in nonionic surfactant
systems.

SELF-DIFFUSION IN SYSTEMS ANALOGOUS TO MICROEMULSIONS

    In the three-component system sodium cholate-decanol-water there
is a single one phase region extending from pure decanol to pure water
and in the system sodium octanoate-octanoic acid-water from water-free
mixtures of acid and soap to more than 96% water. The self-diffusion
coefficients of all the components were determined for these systems
as a function of sample composition[30]. In both cases, and in particular for the latter system, there is a quite regular and feature-less

variation of the self-diffusion coefficients of all species as one
goes from low to high water concentrations. At intermediate compositions where all three components are present in large amounts all the
self-diffusion coefficients are relatively large. In none of the
systems, at any concentration, one encounters a situation which according to the above discussion should be characteristic of typical normal
or reversed micelles.

VIEWS ON THE STRUCTURE AND DYNAMICS OF MICROEMULSIONS

     For typical microemulsion systems, with ionic or nonionic surfac-
tant, as well as for two "microemulsion analogous" systems we have
observed diffusion coefficients of both hydrophilic and hydrophobic
species to be very high. This should contain significant information
on micro-emulsion structure; one cannot hope to put forward detailed
models, but the diffusion data certainly can exclude certain models in
the literature and give good indications of what the correct model
would look like. Many studies by different physico-chemical methods
have been used for the same problems but it will not be possible to go
into any discussion of this here; in many cases the relation between
observed quantities and structural features is unclear. We will only
mention here two in our opinion very important observations which
perhaps have not been sufficiently considered. Firstly, the viscosities are generally quite low for microemulsions. This seems to rule
out well-defined structures with amphiphile aggregates extending in
one way or another over long distances; typical such structures are
the model of the cubic liquid crystal proposed by Luzzati, [16,17] the
periodic structures proposed by Scriven[34] and the rod-like micellar
solutions. One would expect that such structures under relatively
minor composition changes would have the tendency to separate out as a
distinct phase. Secondly, proton NMR spectra for several systems
investigated show quite narrow lines. Interpretation of NMR relaxation
of amphiphilic systems is complicated by the fact that one has large
slowly moving aggregates within which very rapid local motion exists;
therefore proton NMR data, inter alia, in the literature are incorrec-
tly interpreted for example in terms of "effective correlation times".
The narrow proton NMR lines rule out the presence of extended structures with a well-defined interface (with order parameters even well
below those of liquid crystalline phases). Instead these observations
imply that one has only small aggregates or if extended aggregates
exist, they have a very flexible, "loose" interface.

     Returning to the self-diffusion data, these taken in isolation
can be interpreted in two alternative ways (or a combination of these),
i.e. 1) either the solutions have a bicontinuous (i.e. both water-
and oil-continuous) structure.
2) or the aggregates present have interfaces which are easily deform-
able and flexible and open up on a very short time-scale.

124   B. LINDMAN ET AL.

Partly from the arguments presented above we have become more
inclined to believe that the second alternative comes closer to the
correct description; however, no doubt much more experimental and
theoretical work is needed for this to be verified.

Several structural models of microemulsions have been proposed
and we will mention only a few important studies here. Taupin and co-
workers[35] consider the presence of hard oil and water globules with
a relatively sharp transition between these, Shinoda[8,36] a lamellar
structure with alternating water, amphiphile and hydrocarbon layers,
Talmon and Prager[37] hard randomly arranged hydrophobic and hydrophilic polyhedra, Scriven[34] complex periodic three dimensional net-
works with both hydrocarbon and water continuity while Friberg et al[
propose a random structure with varying curvatures. In these studies,
which have all contributed to our understanding of microemulsions, it
seems (although this is not always clearly stated) that one generally
favours a hard well-defined interface of the type encountered for, for
example, lamellar liquid crystals or micelles.

A condition for the formation of typical microemulsions in
micelle-forming ionic surfactant systems seems to be the presence of a
short-chain alcohol like pentanol or butanol and in order to understan
micro-emulsion structure it is important to consider the effect of the
alcohol on the formation of well-defined interfaces. With a long-chai
alcohol like decanol, with very low aqueous solubility, one obtains in
the center of the phase diagram an extensive region with lamellar
liquid crystal. Unlike decanol, pentanol (or butanol) can partition
between the hydrophobic and hydrophilic domains, and the interface,
with comparable probability. The effect of this can be viewed in
different ways but it seems reasonable that this creation of a much
less distinct hydrophobic-hydrophilic separation strongly facilitates
transport of the different entities over the interface. Expressed
differently, the amphiphile aggregates present should have a very
flexible interface which constantly opens up and reforms. Spectroscopic studies which can monitor such very rapid motion (perhaps in
the nanosecond range) are important to verify these points. As a
conclusion of this discussion we may propose that for typical microemulsions there is

a) a polydispersity in aggregate size and shape;
b) very rapid changes in aggregate size and shape;
c) a relatively low order at the hydrophilic-hydrophobic interface.

Very similar ideas on different aspects discussed above have been
put forward in recent most significant studies by Eicke[38,39]
Bostock et al[33] and Zana[40]; these authors have other starting
points for their discussion and express their views in alternative
ways but it seems that one approaches a common view on many important
points. As regards microemulsion dynamics the recent review paper by
Zana and Lang[40] contains much significant information. In kinetic

studies one demonstrates directly that the presence of a short chain
alcohol accelerates considerably the exchange of surfactant between
different domains. These authors also give evidence for a very rapid
fusion and fisson of aggregates in microemulsion solutions and conclude that very labile structures are present.

FUTURE PROSPECTS OF THE SELF-DIFFUSION STUDIES. THE FOURIER
TRANSFORM NMR DIFFUSION METHOD FOR COMPLEX SYSTEMS

It is our belief that the self-diffusion studies can give information on structure and dynamics of amphiphilic systems, not the least
for complex systems where many other techniques are difficult to apply.
The investigations reported on above were performed with two different
complementary experimental approaches, i.e. the open-ended capillary
tube method employing radioactive labelling and the NMR pulsed gradient spin-echo method with ^{1}H or ^{2}H NMR; experimental details are given
elsewhere[32]. These methods have both advantages and limitations.
The capillary tube method can be used for very low concentrations for
almost any entity, but is slow and not applicable for highly viscous
systems and above all the radioactive labelling required can be
extremely difficult and involve time-consuming synthetic work. The
NMR method is very rapid, has a relatively high sensitivity in proton
NMR but often requires that protons in all but one component are
exchanged to deuterons, an impossible task in most cases; deuteron
NMR has important sensitivity limitations. With this background it
was of very great interest to us that Stilbs and Moseley[41-43]
recently developed the Fourier transform pulsed gradient spin-echo
NMR technique for a standard NMR spectrometer. With this technique
it is possible to simultaneously monitor the translational motion of
a large number of species in a microemulsion or any other complex
system using either ^{1}H or ^{13}C NMR; one is somewhat limited as regards
very low diffusion coefficients but this seems to be no significant
limitation for microemulsions. Studies are in progress using the FT
NMR technique in both ^{1}H and ^{13}C NMR and the results confirm and
extend to many other microemulsion systems the conclusions given
above[44,45].

ACKNOWLEDGEMENTS

B. Lindman has received project and travel grants from the
Swedish Natural Sciences Research Council and his stays in Montpellier
were supported by the Centre National de la Recherche Scientifique.
We acknowledge also helpful comments on this work by Håkan Wennerström,
Gordon J. T. Tiddy, Kozo Shinoda and Raoul Zana.

REFERENCES

1. K. Shinoda and S. Friberg, Adv. Colloid Interface Sci., $\underline{4}$, 281,
    (1975).
2. S. Friberg in "Microemulsions", L. M. Prince, ed., Academic Press,
    New York, 133, (1977).

3. S. Friberg, I. Lapczynska and G. Gillberg, J. Colloid Interface
    Sci., 56, 19, (1976).
4. P. Ekwall, Adv. Liquid Cryst., 1, 1, (1975).
5. H. Wennerström and B. Lindman, Phys. Reports, 52, 1, (1979).
6. B. Lindman and H. Wennerström, Topics in Current Chemistry, 87,
    1, (1980).
7. L. M. Prince, ed, "Microemulsions", Academic Press, New York,
    (1977).
8. K. Shinoda and H. Saito, J. Colloid Interface Sci., 26, 70, (196{
9. G. Gillberg, H. Lehtinen, and S. Friberg, J. Colloid Interface
    Sci., 33, 40, (1970).
10. P. Ekwall and L. Mandell, Kolloid Z. Z. Polym., 233, 938, (1969).
11. K. Fontell, Kolloid Z. Z. Polym., 250, 825 (1972).
12. H. Wennerström, B. Lindman, O. Söderman, T. Drakenberg and
    J. B. Rosenholm, J. Amer. Chem. Soc., 101, 6860, (1979).
13. B. Lindman and H. Wennerström in "Solution Chemistry of Surfact-
    ants", E. J. Fendler and K. L. Mittal, eds., Plenum Press, New
    York, in press.
14. G. Lindblom and H. Wennerström, Biophys. Chem., 6, 167, (1977).
15. T. Bull and B. Lindman, Mol. Cryst. Liq. Cryst. 28, 155, (1975).
16. K. Fontell in "Liquid Crystals and Plastic Crystals", Vol. 2,
    G. W. Gray and P. A. Winsor, eds., Ellis Horwood Publishers,
    Chichester, U.K., 80, 1974.
17. A. Tardieu and V. Luzzati, Biochim. Biophys. Acta 219, 11, (1970)
18. V. Luzzati and P. A. Spegt, Nature 215, 701, (1967).
19. V. Luzzati, A. Tardieu, T. Gulik-Kryzwicki, E. Rivas, and
    F. Reiss-Husson, Nature, 220, 485, (1968).
20. V. Luzzati, T. Gulik-Krzywicki, and A. Tardieu, Nature, 217,
    1028, (1968).
21. G. W. Gray and P. A. Winsor, Mol. Cryst. Liq. Cryst. 26, 305,
    (1974).
22. D. Coates and G. W. Gray, The Microscope, 24, 117, (1976).
23. P. A. Winsor, Symposia Farada Soc., no 5, 1971 pp 89 and 161
    (1972).
24. G. W. Gray and P. A. Winsor in "Liquid Crystals and Plastic
    Crystals", G. W. Gray and P. A. Winsor, eds., Horwood, Chichester
    U.K., vol. 1., 1, (1974).
25. J. Charvolin and A. Tardieu in "Liquid Crystals", L. Liebert,
    ed., Solid State Physics Suppl., 14, 209, (1978).
26. G. Lindblom, K. Larsson, L. Johansson, K. Fontell and S. Forsén,
    J. Amer. Chem. Soc., 101, 5465, (1979).
27. N. Kamenka, B. Lindman and B. Brun, Colloid Polym. Sci., 252,
    144, (1974).
28. J. Clifford and B. A. Pethica, Trans. Faraday Soc., 60, 216,
    (1964).
29. J. Clifford and B. A. Pethica, J. Phys. Chem. 70, 3345, (1966).
30. H. Fabre, Thesis, Montpellier, 1980. H. Fabre, N. Kamenka and
    B. Lindman, to be published.
31. Å. Johansson and B. Lindman in "Liquid Crystals and Plastic
    Crystals", G. W. Gray and P. A. Winsor, eds., Horwood,
    Chichester, U.K., 1974, vol. 2, 195.

32.   B. Lindman, N. Kamenka, T.-M. Kathopoulis, B. Brun and
      P.-G. Bilsson, J. Phys. Chem., 84, 2485 (1980).
33.   T. A. Bostock, M. P. McDonald, G. J. T. Tiddy and L. Waring, to
      be published.
34.   L. E. Scriven in "Micellization, Solubilization, and Micro-
      emulsions"., K. L. Mittal, ed., Plenum Press, New York, vol. 2.,
      877, (1977).
35.   M. Lagües. R. Ober and C. Taupin, J. de Physique Lettres, 39, 487,
      (1978).
36.   H. Saito and K. Shinoda, J. Colloid Interface Sci., 32, 647,
      (1970).
37.   Y. Talmon and S. Prager, J. Chem. Phys., 69, 517, (1978).
38.   M. Zulauf and H._F. Eicke, J. Phys. Chem., 83, 480, (1979).
39.   H.-F. Eicke, Pure Appl. Chem., 52, 1349, (1980).
40.   R. Zana and J. Lang in "Solution Chemistry of Surfactants",
      E. J. Fendler and K. L. Mittal, eds., Plenum Press, New York,
      in press.
41.   P. Stilbs and M. E. Moseley, Chem. Scripta 13, 26, (1979).
42.   P. Stilbs and M. E. Moseley, Chem. Scripta, 15, 176 (1980).
43.   M. E. Moseley and P. Stilbs, Chem. Scripta, 15, 215 (1980).
44.   P. Stilbs, M. E. Moseley and B. Lindman, J. Magn. Resonance, 40,
      401 (1980).
45.   M. E. Moseley, P. Stilbs and B. Lindman, to be published.

DISCUSSION

Dr. A. Höhener: Do the diffusion results from the tracer method and
NMR agree? There is, for example, a lot of difficulty to get agreement in plastic phases.

Prof. B. Lindman: One would anticipate that tracer and NMR self-
diffusion should agree and indeed they do for the several cases where
we have done both types of measurements. For the case of separation
into very extended domains (of the order of $10^4 - 10^5$ Å) the very
different effective diffusion times come into play. Then it is possible to observe restricted diffusion phenomena by NMR, which has been
done for suspensions of cells.

Our tracer technique is not applicable for highly viscous systems
and therefore we have no experience of plastic phases.

Prof. F. Franks: In the system H_2O-Na octanoate-decanol $D/_Do$ for
water increases rapidly as the surfactant concentration approaches
100% while $D/_Do$ for the other components remains constant. How is
this interpreted?

Prof. B. Lindman: $D/_Do$ for both water and sodium ions increases at
the highest decanol contents. This is interpreted in terms of the
presence of reversed micelles with water cores containing the counterions at lower decanol contents. The partial confinement of water and
counterions in the water cores leads to slow diffusion over large

distances. At high decanol contents the reversed micelles break down
and this confinement becomes eliminated. Then the kinetic entities
are smaller, for example free (solvated) water molecules or ions or
ion-pairs.

Dr J. E. Crooks: (i) Do you believe that rapid partitioning of the
short chain alcohol is an essential feature of microemulsion stability
Region L_1 in the octanoic acid/decanol/water system is a microemulsion
where the decanol acts as a short chain alcohol linked to an alkane.
(ii) Do you see a difference in type between systems such as the
octanoate/decanol/water system in which there is a lamellar liquid
crystal phase in between the O/W and W/O phases, and those in which
there is a continuous range of isotropic solution from O/W to W/O?
Would you think of the latter as "true" microemulsions?

Prof. B. Lindman: (i) A short-chain alcohol like butanol or pentanol
is firstly distributed to a great extent over both hydrophilic and
hydrophobic domains and over internal interfaces and secondly it considerably decreases the lifetime of the surfactant in the interfaces.
This is beclieved to be typical of the four-component "co-surfactant"
type microemulsions. With a long-chain alcohol like decanol these
features are not present leading to quite different solution structure
and phase diagrams. It seems not possible to approximate the effect
of decanol as the sum of a short-chain alcohol and an alkane. (ii)
This difference is indeed quite marked as discussed in the paper.
With the present confusion as regards the nomenclature it is not possi
ble to say what is a "true" microemulsion. It seems very important to
establish the structure of the solutions for different microemulsion
systems.

Prof. H. T. Davies: Why do you believe there are very many small
aggregates in microemulsions? Do you imagine these aggregates as
dynamic objects, flickering with high frequency into and out of being
throughout the system?

Prof. B. Lindman: Firstly, it has been demonstrated by Zana and Lang
(ref. 40 of the paper) that the presence of a short-chain alcohol
considerably reduces the lifetime of a surfactant monomer in a micelle
Surfactant association being diffusion-controlled this leads to the
result that the alcohol reduces aggregate size. Secondly, it has been
demonstrated that a short-chain alcohol is distributed rather equally
between micelles and intermicellar solution (P. Stilbs, J. Colloid
Interface Sci., in press). Furthermore, the viscosity of microemulsions is generally quite small and transverse proton magnetic relaxation is slow; both these observations exclude the presence of extended
aggregates. Finally, the self diffusion studies demonstrate a high
mobility of all components, which is consistent with the presence of
small aggregates.

Prof. J. Th G. Overbeek: Why do you plot $D/_{D}o$ - it must be remembered the pure decanol is quite viscous?

Prof. B. Lindman: This criticism is certainly relevant. The reason for doing so was that the molecular mobility depends on several factors molecular interactions, confinement into domains and mere molecular size effects. The latter are uninteresting in the present context and should best be accounted for separately. This is certainly not trivial and the method used by us has problems for example as you imply in pure decanol there is a strong self-association due to hydrogen-bonding. The best way to obtain D^O would probably be to measure the self-diffusion coefficients of all components in an inert non-associating solvent. This has, however, not been done, and is not easy to do.

PHASE DIAGRAM AND INTERFACIAL TENSIONS OF BRINE-DODECANE-PENTANOL-SODIUM OCTYLBENZENESULFONATE SYSTEM

A.M. Bellocq, J. Biais, P. Bothorel, D. Bourbon, B. Clin,
P. Lalanne, B. Lemanceau

Centre de Recherche Paul Pascal-Domaine Universitaire
33405 Talence Cedex
France

INTRODUCTION

This system has been chosen as a typical model in the frame of research on microemulsions and their use in tertiary oil recovery. The phase diagrams of such systems present one-phase, two-phase, three-phase regions. The needs of tertiary oil recovery lead to try to find out active mixtures (surfactants and cosurfactants) able to dissolve large amounts of oil and water and to achieve low interfacial tensions. The very low interfacial tensions are generally observed on three-phase states such as an intermediary (middle) phase (m) is in equilibrium with an aqueous phase (w) and an organic phase (o). Such states are called of Winsor's type III. It exists conditions to observe the equality of interfacial tensions γ_{mw} and γ_{mo}; these conditions have been termed optimal (see e.g. 1-7).

The purpose of this study is to explore the phase behaviour of the mentioned system and to examine the relationships between interfacial tensions and concentrations. We report new results both on multi-phase behaviour and interfacial properties: it can exist several types of three-phase states; more over the possibility to observe a crossing of the interfacial tensions curves when a parameter is varied depends on the path of variation of the parameter.

EXPERIMENTAL SECTION

Samples preparations have been made with components of high purity and the measurements achieved at constant temperature (21°C) after sufficient storage time at this temperature. The one-phase regions boundaries have been determined by turbidity point method and

the concentrations in the various phases by chromatography or NMR.
The interfacial tensions have been measured by the spinning drop meth
with the Clausthal University apparatus (W. Germany). The concentration are expressed in weight percentage.

EXPERIMENTAL RESULTS

1. Phase diagrams

    We have chosen to show the more significant sections of the space
of the diagram representation.

    Preliminary study of the water-pentanol-OBS (octyl benzene sul-
fonate) system shows a large one-phase region (true ternary system)
Fig. 1a.

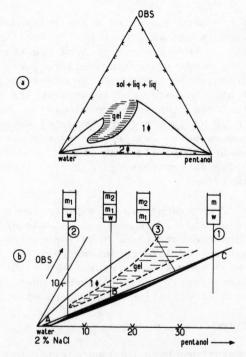

Fig.1. (a), (b) pseudoternary diagrams (weight percent) at 24°C of
the sodium p.octylbenzene sulfonate (OBS)-pentanol-water and 2% NaCl
water. m_1, m_2 = micellar solutions; w = aqueous phase

Addition of NaCl up to 2% reduces the one-phase region and produces the appearance of a three-phase region, Fig. 1b. The three-phase state is formed by an aqueous phase in equilibrium with two micellar phases. The concentrations of the components in the various phases are practically the same whatever may be the overall concentration (Table I). This state is very close to a three-phase state of a true ternary system.

Sections of the diagram of the five components system at fixed water salinity and fixed alcohol/surfactant ratio (A/S) are shown on Fig. 2. In absence of salt the region below the demixing line is a two-phase one comprising a microemulsion in equilibrium with an oil phase; this state is termed Winsor's type I. Addition of salt first causes the demixing line to be lowered, the appearance of a second two-phase region characterized by an equilibrium between an aqueous phase and microemulsion (Winsor's type II) and a three-phase region characterized by an equilibrium between an oil phase and two microemulsions. Increasing salinity up to 2% two new three-phase regions appear; the one is located in the water rich region, the other much larger is of Winsor's type III. We want to bring particularly our attention on this state. Figs 2c and 2d show the effect of varying the A/S ratio at constant water salinity; Fig. 3 more precisely shows the effect of this ratio on the extension of the type III region. The effect of increasing this ratio is qualitatively the same than increasing salinity.

2.   Concentrations in polyphasic region

We have measured the concentrations in several phases in equilibrium, following two paths in the representation space: the both paths at constant water salinity 2% and constant water/oil ratio (WOR : 4,5); the first path is characterized by the ratio A/S = 2, the second one by A/S = 5; the variable parameter is the sum A + S (active mixture). .

Fig. 4 show the concentrations in the microemulsion phase along these two paths. As the change I $\longrightarrow$ III $\longrightarrow$ II occurs, the water content of the microemulsion decreases while the oil content increases. The magnitude of these variations are much larger along the second path.

Fig. 5 show the concentrations in the aqueous and organic phases; these concentrations small change although the concentrations of water and oil in microemulsion middle phase change in a large extent. Whatever the state of the system is (I, III or II) surfactant is concentrated in the microemulsion phase.

3.   Interfacial tensions (Fig. 6)

We have measured several interfacial tensions along the two above mentioned paths that is to say: γ_{wm} of type I, γ_{wm}, γ_{mo} and γ_{ow} of

TABLE I

Compositions of Phases in the System OBS, Pentanol, H_2O, 2% NaCl

	I			II		
	OBS	C_5OH	H_2O	OBS	C_5OH	H_2O
Overall Composition	3	7	90*	8	16	76*
Lower Phase	/	1.65	98.35	/	1.5	98.5
Middle Phase	4.6	8.7	86.7	4.6	10	85.4
Upper Phase	11.1	24.15	64.75	12.9	23.9	63.2

* H_2O, NaCl 20g/l.

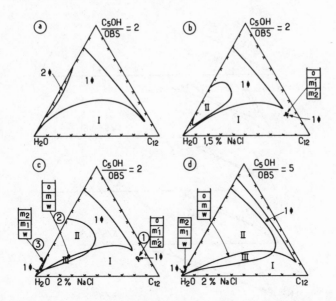

Fig.2. Pseudoternary diagrams (weight percent) at 24°C of the sodium p.octyl-benzene sulfonate (OBS)-pentanol-water-dodecane at various salinities and active mixture compositions. (a) C_5OH/OBS = 2 - 0% NaCl; (b) C_5OH/OBS = 2 - 1,5% NaCl; (c) C_5OH/OBS = 2 - 2% NaCl; (d) C_5OH/OBS = 5 - 2% NaCl; m_1', m_2', m_1, m_2 = microemulsion phases, o = organic phase, w = aqueous phase.

type III and γ_{mo} of type II. The main trends are the following; as the active mixture increases γ_{wm} increases when γ_{mo} decreases; the lowest tensions (10^{-2} to 10^{-3} m N/m) are observed in the three phase region; in this region the γ_{wm} and γ_{mo} curves are crossing along the second path, but not along the first one; in this region γ_{ow} is always larger than the sum $\gamma_{wm} + \gamma_{mo}$, but its value is low.

DISCUSSION

This system with brine, oil, surfactant and alcohols is a five component system and needs a four-dimensional space to be described at constant temperature and pressure. We have treated these systems at constant water salinity in the pseudo-quaternary system approximation, the brine being a pseudo component; the system may be described in a three dimensional space. In this approximation at constant temperature and pressure the two-phase state is bivariant: the concentrations of the phases in equilibrium are described by the ends of tie-lines; these ends are located on corresponding elements of

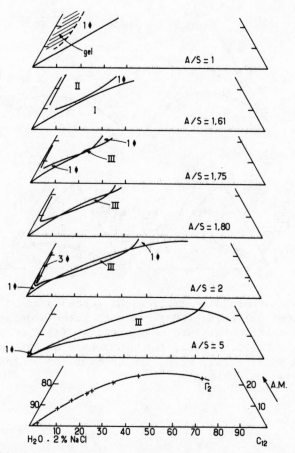

Fig. 3. Pseudoternary diagrams defined by various A/S ratios,
salinity = 2% NaCl. The lower curve (Γ_2 curve) is the locus of the
projections of the points connecting the one- and three-phase regions
on the water-alcohol-oil plane.

demixing surface. The tie lines do not generally lie in the plane
defined by constant A/S. Along a linear path through a two-phase
region, the phase concentrations describe two curves on demixing
surfaces; these curves depend on the path.

The three-phase state is monovariant; the concentrations of the
phases are defined by three corresponding points M_1, M_2, M_3 describing
the curve Γ_1, Γ_2 Γ_3; these curve elements are located on demixing surface. The three-phase volume in the representation space is generated
by the continuous stacking of the tie triangles such as M_1 M_2 M_3

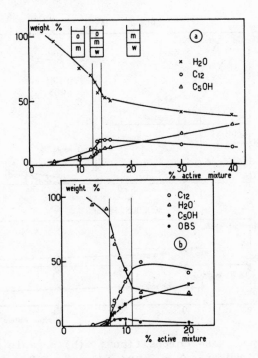

Fig.4. Microemulsion phase compositions;
a) mixtures defined by A/S=2, WOR=4,5, salinity - 2% NaCl as a function of the active mixture content in the overall system; T = 21°C.
b) mixtures defined by A/S = 5, WOR=4,5, salinity = 2% NaCl.

(fig 7). The intersection of this volume with a plane corresponding
to a given A/S ratio defines the three-phase region in this plane
(limited by the curve (aC'bC on the fig. 7). If the plane under study
intercept the Γ_2 curve in two points, these points belonging to the
one-phase region, the three-phase region is connected by these two
points to the single phase one. It is the case in this study; projection of the Γ_2 curve is shown on fig. 3.

     The use of this pseudoquaternary representation is the following:
the concentrations of the microemulsion phase are practically described by the Γ_2 curve. This approximation is then justified. Moreover,
the figs 3 and 7 show that the concentrations in the middle phase are
always included in the segment CC'. This explains why the crossing
of the water and oil concentration curves only appears along the
second path (A/S=S). The parts of Γ_2 described are limited by WOR 1,3
and 11,5 for A/S=2 and by WOR 0.25 and 39 for A/S=5.

     In the same way in this approximation, the interfacial tensions
in the three-phase region depend on only one concentration parameter

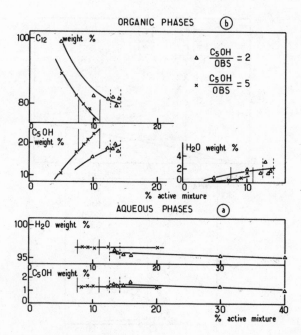

Fig.5. (a) Aqueous phase compositions; (b) organic phase compositions for mixtures defined by A/S = 2 and A/S = 5, WOR = 4,5, salinity - 2% NaCl as a function of the active mixture content in the overall system

in one of the phases, for instance the water content in the middle phase. Fig. 8 shows the variations of γ_{wm} and γ_{mo} as a function of the water content in the middle phase: whatever the path is, the γ_{ij} values are practically the same in the region belonging to the two paths. As it exists in the three-phase state relations between concentrations of one component belonging to two phases, it also exists relations between γ_{ij} values and the difference between concentrations of water (or oil) in middle phase and aqueous phase (or middle phase and oil phase) (fig 9). For instance, γ_{mw} is all the more smaller as the difference of the water content is smaller; then the system approaches a critical end point. The Γ_2 curve is specific of the investigated system: in general case the equality of the water and oil contents of microemulsion does not coincide with the equality of interfacial tension γ_{wm} and γ_{mo}.

It is worthwhile to notice that the variation of a given property of one of the phase is continuous along a path through boundary between the two phase and the three phase region, but slope is discontinuous as shown for instance the refractive index curve of the middle phase along the second path (Fig.10).

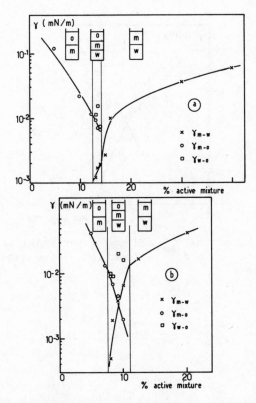

Fig.6. Interfacial tensions for (a) mixtures defined by A/S = 2,
WOR = 4,5, salinity - 2% NaCl. (b) mixtures defined by A/S = 5,
WOR = 4,5 salinity = 2% NaCl as a function of the active mixture
content in the overall system; T = 21°C.

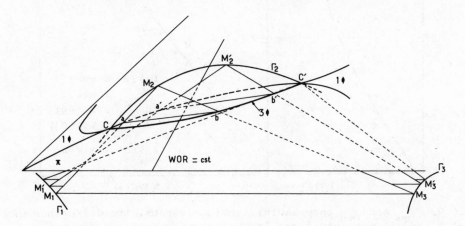

Fig.7. Section of the three-phase volume with a π plane.

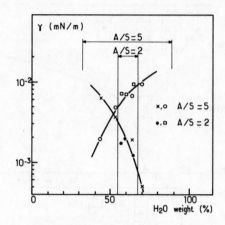

Fig.8. Dependence of the γ_{mw} and γ_{mo} interfacial tensions in the planes $A/S = 2$ and $A/S = 5$ as a function of the water weight percentage in the middle phase.

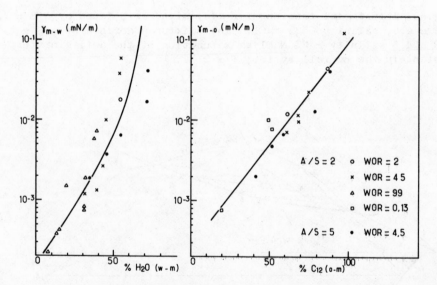

Fig.9. γ_{mw} and γ_{mo} interfacial tensions versus, the difference of water and oil concentrations in the considered phases (w = aqueous phase, m = microemulsion phase, o = organic phase) for the systems defined by $A/S = 2$, WOR = 4,5 and 99: $A/S = 5$, WOR = 4,5.

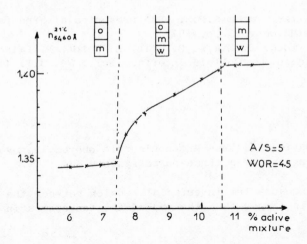

Fig.10. Refractive index of microemulsion phase versus the overall active mixture concentration along the path: WOR ≒ 4,5; A/OBS = 5; water salinity 2%.

CONCLUSION

The phase behaviour of studied system is quite similar to that previously reported for the brine-toluene-butanol-SOS system (8) and similar to those reported by Salter (6). Moreover our data show that conditions which promote middle phase microemulsion formation do not always lead to a crossing of the interfacial tension curves. Whatever the path followed in the three-phase region is, it exists one single relationship between the value of the interfacial tension γ_{mw} (or γ_{mo}) and one variable of composition in one of the phases. Phase analysis point that the water-oil pair in the middle phase is close to a state analogous to a critical one. This result has certainly to be related to the very low interfacial tensions observed.

REFERENCES

1. R. N. Healy, R. L. Reed and D. G. Stenmark, S.P.E. Journal, 16, 147, (1976).
2. W. Wade, J. C. Morgan, R. S. Schechter, J. K. Jacobson and J. L. Salager, Paper S.P.E. 6844, presented at 52nd fall meeting of S.P.E.-AIME, Denver, 1977.
3. J. L. Salager, E. Vasquez, J. C. Morgan, R. S. Schechter and W. H. Wade, Paper S.P.E. 7054 presented at 5th S.P.E. symposium on improved oil recovery, Tulsa, 1978.
4. S. C. Jones and K. D. Dreher, S.P.E. Journal 16, 161, (1976).
5. W. C. Hsieh and D. O. Shah, Paper S.P.E. 6594 presented at SPE-AIME Symposium on oilfield and geothermal chemistry La Jolla, Ca. 1977.

6. S. J. Salter, Paper S.P.E. 6843 presented at 52nd fall meeting
    of SPE-AIME Denver, Co. 1977.
7. A. M. Bellocq, J. Biais, B. Clin, B. Gelot, P. Lalanne and
    B. Lemanceau, J. Colloid Interface Sci., 74, 311, (1980).

DISCUSSION

Prof H. T. Davis: (i) Was Antonov's rule obeyed whenever you measured
the three tensions of a three-phase system?

Prof B. Lemanceau: The interfacial tension between the lower and
upper phase is larger than the sum of the two others in the three-
phase region.

Prof H. T. Davis: It is thermodynamically disallowed that $\gamma_{ow} > \gamma_{om}$
+ γ_{wm} unless there is so little of some component in the oil and
water rich phases that a thin film of microemulsion cannot form without depleting the oil and water rich phases of that component. What
is thermodynamically allowed is the triangle inequality.

$$\gamma_{ow} < \gamma_{om} + \gamma_{wm}$$

Violation of this inequality could arise from lack of chemical
equilibrium or temperature drift in the tensiometer. We have traced
some such violations to temperature drift in our spinning drop tensio-
metry of alcohol-brine-hydrocarbon systems.

Prof M. Kahlweit: Antonov's rule is not a fundamental thermodynamic
principle. It is also difficult to measure the 3 surface tensions
accurately enough. Are they temperature dependent?

Prof B. Lemanceau: The interfacial tensions are certainly temperature
dependent. We have kept the temperature constant within the limit of
0.1^{o}C.

Dr. I. D. Robb: The interdependency of the two interfacial tensions
requires brine being one component. This would not be the case if
there were preferential hydration of certain regions or the water and
salt were not identically distributed between the phases.

Prof B. Lemanceau: The salinity is practically the same in the lower
phase and the middle phase; increasing the active content from 8 to
12.44% (on path 2) the salinity lies between 1.9 and 2.1% in the lower
phase and 1.9 to 2.2% in the middle phase. The upper phase only
contains a very small amount of water.

ALCOHOL EFFECTS ON TRANSITIONS IN LIQUID

CRYSTALLINE DISPERSIONS

P. K. Kilpatrick, F. D. Blum, H. T. Davis, A. H. Falls,
E. W. Kaler, W. G. Miller, J. E. Puig, L. E. Scriven,
Y. Talmon and N. A. Woodbury

Departments of Chemical Engineering and Materials Science
and of Chemistry
University of Minnesota
Minneapolis, Minnesota 55455

INTRODUCTION

A surfactant can be defined as an amphiphilic compound that forms fluid microstructures with both polar and non-polar solvents. A single-tail surfactant with a straight-chain hydrophobic moiety of sufficient length forms micelles in water above a characteristic range of concentrations called the critical micelle concentration. Double-tail surfactants form micelles only when their hydrophobic chains are sufficiently short[1]. Naturally occurring double-tail surfactants such as lecithins separate in a lamellar liquid crystalline phase in aqueous solution as concentration is increased. Synthetic double-tail surfactants have also been found to form lamellar liquid crystals at low concentrations in water. Both double- and single-tail surfactants form microemulsions when combined in certain proportions with water, hydrocarbons, and, often, salts and alcohols or other cosolvents. By microemulsion we mean a thermodynamically stable, microstructured fluid phase of variable composition that incorporates substantial amounts of oil, water and surfactants[2]. With some nonionic surfactant systems, neither alcohols nor added electrolytes are necessary in the formulation of a microemulsion[3,4]. However, most ionic surfactant-oil-water systems form stable nonequilibrium macroemulsions in the absence of alcohols or added salts. In all likelihood, these emulsions are stabilized by viscous liquid crystalline or mesomorphic films of low interfacial tension encapsulating the emulsion droplets[5]. Salts moderate the long-range forces produced by the electrical double layers of the ionic surfactant head groups. The role of alcohols is not clear, although they probably serve as viscosity

143

depressants by solvating the surfactant molecules and thus reducing
regions of high local surfactant concentration such as are present in
mesomorphic phases. Further work is clearly needed to elucidate the
mechanisms responsible for stabilizing and destabilizing macroemulsions in microemulsion-forming systems.

Our goal is to find the effect of low molecular weight alcohols
(t-butanol, n-butanol, n-pentanol, and n-hexanol) on lamellar liquid
crystalline dispersions of a model double-tail surfactant in aqueous
solution and to determine the resulting microstructures. The surfactant chosen for study, sodium 4-(1'-heptylnonyl)benzenesulfonate
(SHBS), was available in relatively pure form and is a representative
of petroleum sulfonates, which are employed in chemical flooding
schemes for enhancing oil recovery. The effect of alcohol on the
microstructure of these aqueous surfactant solutions likely determines
the resulting microstructure when oil is added.

EXPERIMENTAL

Materials: Water was drawn through a four-stage Millipore cartridge
system. Its conductivity was lower than 1 μS/cm. It was stored in
polyethylene bottles to eliminate leaching of ions, which occurs from
glass containers[6,7]. The alcohols were either Fisher Scientific
A.C.S. pure grade, Mallinckrodt or Aldrich products.

The surfactant SHBS (referred to alternatively in other publications as "Texas #1" and SPHS) was synthesized at the University of
Texas at Austin under a Department of Energy contract to
R. S. Schechter and W. H. Wade. It was purified as described
previously[6,7] and was stored under vacuum in a dessicator over
$CaCl_2$. The surfactant sodium dodecylsulfate (SDS) was obtained in
very pure form (>99 wt %) from BDH, Poole, England and was used without further purification. Solutions of SDS were prepared immediately
before use to minimize hydrolysis of dodecylsulfate ions.

The decane was either an Aldrich Gold Label or a Phillips product
both 99+ mole % pure. The hydrocarbon was stored in glass and used
without further purification. The sodium chloride was Fisher
Scientific certified A.C.S. product and was dried immediately before
use.

Methods: Turbidity was measured with a Cary 15 UV-visible recording,
double-beam spectrophotometer. Quartz cuvettes with 1-cm pathlengths
were used.

Conductances were measured with a Brinkmann E518 Series 4
conductometer. A Jones-type cell with a cell constant of 6.76 cm^{-1}
was used. Electrode polarization effects at low frequency and
low conductances for a given cell constant are peculiar to the
conductometer design and had to be avoided. Samples were

temperature-controlled at $25.00 \pm 0.02°C$ in a water bath using a
Lauda model B-1 heating circulator.

NMR ^{13}C and ^{23}Na spectra were taken on a Varian XL-100 spectrometer operating in the FT mode at 25.2 MHz for the ^{13}C nucleus and
26.5 MHz for the ^{23}Na nucleus. Chemical shifts were measured relative
to a solution of sodium tetraphenyl boron in CD_3CN for ^{23}Na. No
internal reference was used for the ^{13}C nucleus. All spectra were
taken at $25° \pm 2°C$.

Transmission electron micrographs were taken on a JEOL JEM-100CX
electron microscope at an accelerating voltage of 100 kV. A special
cold-stage module, developed by Talmon et al[8,9], was used to transfer fast-frozen hydrated samples into the microscope.

X-ray scattering measurements were made with two different x-ray
cameras in order to explore two ranges of the magnitude of the scat-
tering vector $s = \frac{2 \sin\theta}{\lambda}$. Here 2θ is the angle between the incident and scattered beams and λ is the radiation wavelength. A
modified Kratky camera was used for s between 1.0×10^{-3} and $2.5 \times$
10^{-2} A^{-1}. A conventional Warhaus pinhole film camera was also used
for s greater than 1.8×10^{-2} A^{-1}. The radiation source for both
was nickel-filtered Cu K_α.

The Kratky camera was modified by the addition of an extended
flight path to incorporate a one-dimensional position sensitive
x-ray detector as described by Russell et al.[10]. The sealed, metal
wire anode detector (a TEC model 210) was filled with a 70% Xe and
30% CH_4 mixture at 220 kPa. Output from the detector was stored in
a multichannel analyzer and data were subsequently manipulated with
a PDP 11/60 computer. Specimen solutions were enclosed in a stainless
steel cell with two thin Mylar windows and thermostatted at $25.0 \pm$
$0.1°C$ during the experiment.

After each experiment the data were corrected for background
scattering by subtracting the scattering observed from a blank cell,
and for any variations in the detector sensitivity. The data were
corrected for the effect of the slit collimation of the Kratky camera
by the method of Schmidt[11]. The scattering pattern in the Warhaus
camera was recorded on Kodak No-screen x-ray film and developed
following the manufacturer's specifications.

RESULTS AND DISCUSSION

Turbid dispersions of SHBS in water were biphasic systems of
spherulitic particles of a lamellar liquid crystal ranging in size
from fractions of microns to tens of microns dispersed in a homogeneous surfactant-saturated, aqueous phase with the surfactant
apparently molecularly dispersed at a concentration of about 0.06 wt %.
The dispersed particles were fairly stable, the smaller ones remaining

suspended for months [6,7]. Knowledge of the state of aggregation of surfactant below its solubility limit in water is important in considering microstructure in SHBS-water-alcohol systems. No conclusive evidence of micelle formation has been found in the binary system SHBS-water in the temperature range 10°C to 90°C. However, Magid[12] has conductimetric evidence of non-Nernstian behaviour below the solubility limit at 45°C. Benton et al.[13] and Puig et al.[14] also have conductimetric evidence that the surfactant may be associating below its solubility limit. The data are not indicative of micellization but may reflect small aggregate formation.

The separating lamellar phase in biphasic SHBS-water dispersions consisted of about 25 wt % water as determined by isopiestic vapour sorption experiments[6,7]. Addition of sufficient alcohol to these turbid dispersions yielded an optically clear isotropic fluid phase. Here by isotropic we mean that there was no evidence of mesomorphic phases as indicated by birefringence or NMR line-broadening. We report here the mechanism whereby alcohol converted the liquid crystalline dispersion to this isotropic phase and the determination of the resulting microstructure. We investigated the effect of the addition of the following alcohols to these dispersions: t-butanol (TBA), isobutanol, sec-butanol, n-butanol (NBA), and n-pentanol (NAA), and n-hexanol (NHA).

Spectroturbidimetry

Turbidity provides one method of determining the phase boundary in passing from biphasic dispersion to an isotropic phase. By measuring the apparent absorbance of incident monochromatic light traversing the sample and subtracting the absorbance due to water, we determined the attenuation due to scattering of the incident light beam. Fig. 1 shows a typical plot of absorbance due to scattering versus wavelength for some SHBS-TBA systems. By fixing the concentration of SHBS in the aqueous dispersion and varying only the amount of TBA added, one determines the TBA/SHBS weight ratio at which the solution becomes isotropic, i.e. clear. Our criterion for spectrophotometric clarity was as absorbance due to scattering at 600 nm less than 0.1. For systems for which this requirement is met, the wavelength dependence cannot be determined due to the large random error in measuring these low absorbances. In Fig. 1, this level was reached for a TBA/SHBS (w/w) of about 6. By taking various wt % SHBS dispersions in water and titrating to clarity with TBA, one can construct a partial ternary phase diagram delineating the binodal that separates the two phase dispersion from the isotropic phase. Fig. 2 shows the alcohol-SHBS-water phase boundary determined by turbidimetry for NBA, TBA, and NAA. For a fixed SHBS/water ratio, the alcohol concentration needed for clearing increased in the order NAA, NBA, TBA. This trend can be rationalized by considering the partition coefficients of these alcohols between water and an oleic phase. NAA partitions preferentially into the lamellar phase and solubilizes the liquid crystals at lower total

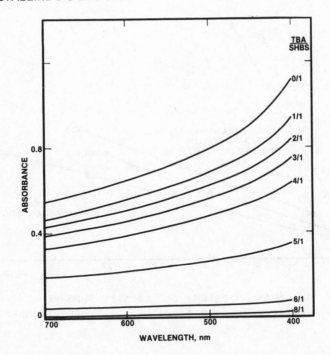

Fig. 1. Absorbance due to scattering versus wavelength for 0.5 wt %
SHBS aqueous solutions with added t-butanol (TBA).

concentration of added alcohol. The process of solubilization refers
here, and below, to the transformation of the dispersed lamellar phase
into the aqueous isotropic phase by the action of alcohol. Thus, the
relative lipophilicity of an added alcohol is an index to its effici-
ency in solubilizing the lamellar phase. Conductimetric and NMR data
confirm this trend.

Conductimetry

    The specific conductivity of aqueous dispersions of SHBS was
measured as a function of added alcohol. The data for TBA are plotted
in Fig. 3 for various wt % SHBS dispersions. Below the solubility
of SHBS in water (0.06 wt %), the alcohol did not affect the conductivity. Above the solubility, the specific conductivity rose mono-
tonically as the amount of alcohol increased, up to a point beyond
which it remained constant with further alcohol addition.

    The observed trends in specific conductivity can be explained
qualitatively in terms of a simple model. Let us assume that the

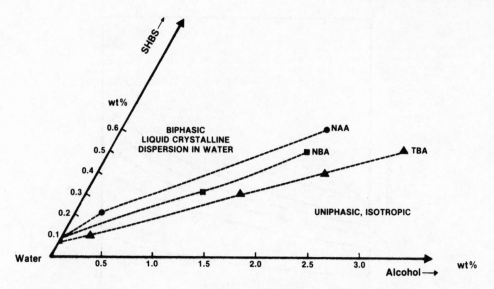

Fig. 2. Partial phase diagrams for ternary SHBS-alcohol-water systems in water-rich corner, as determined by spectroturbidimetry.

liquid crystallites are monodispersed spheres of radius R_c and that all the charge carriers in the system obey Stokes' law, i.e., the mobility of a carrier obeys the equation

$$\zeta = \frac{q}{\alpha\pi\eta R} \qquad \ldots(1)$$

where η is the viscosity of the aqueous solution, q and R the charge and radius of the carrier, and $\alpha = 4$ for carriers of molecular dimensions and $\alpha = 6$ for carriers large on a molecular scale. The charge of a crystallite is $q_c = z\_e(1-f) \, 4\pi R_c^2 \, \sigma$, where f is the fraction of bound counterions at the surface of the crystallite and σ is the surface density of surfactant molecules. The specific conductivity of the dispersion for the model is

$$\kappa = \phi \, \frac{e^2\sigma}{2\pi\eta} \left[(1-f)^2 \, 4\pi\sigma z_-^2 + \frac{3}{2} \, \frac{(1-f)z_+^2}{R_c R_+} \right] + \frac{n_s e^2}{4\pi\eta} \left[\frac{z_+^2}{R_+} + \frac{z_-^2}{R_-} \right] \ldots(2)$$

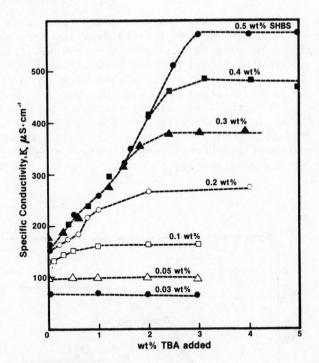

Fig. 3. Specific conductivity versus added t-butanol (TBA) for
various wt % SHBS dispersions in water.

where ϕ is the volume fraction of the crystallites in the dispersion,
n_s is the number density of surfactant in the aqueous solution, e
the unit electronic charge, and z_- and z_+ the valences of sodium and
surfactant ions, respectively. For SHBS, $z_+ = z_- = 1$. Equation (2)
neglects the effects of ionic interactions and association or aggregation of dissolved surfactant, effects that would be significant in
quantitative calculations but will not change the basic trends predicted by this model.

Below the solubility limit (~0.06 wt %) of SHBS, there are no
crystallites so that $\phi = 0$ and n_s is constant; the conductivity
according to Eq. (2) varies as alcohol is added only if the
viscosity changes. Separate viscosity measurements, not reported
here, have shown that the viscosity varies little with addition of
a few percent of alcohol. Thus, the constatn conductivity seen in
Fig. 3 at SHBS levels of 0.03 and 0.05 wt % is explained by Equation (2).
Above the solubility limit, however, ϕ is not zero at zero alcohol
and the conductivity derives from the crystallites, their counterions,

and the dissolved surfactant; that the latter furnishes the major contribution even at 0.5 wt % SHBS follows from the zero alcohol data in
Fig. 3. Addition of alcohol dissolves the crystallites, ϕ going to
zero and n_s increasing to its maximum value at total dissolution of
the crystallites. The gain in conductivity due to increase in dissolved surfactant is much larger than the loss due to dissolution of the
crystallites. Thus, the conductivity increases with addition of
alcohol until all the crystallites are dissolved. It then levels off
because the liquid crystallites are dissolved and n_s remains constant
with further alcohol addition. These trends are again explained by
the model yielding Equation (2).

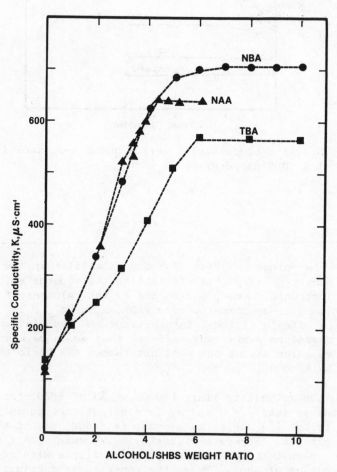

Fig. 4. Specific conductivity versus alcohol/SHBS weight ratio for
0.5 wt % SHBS solutions with added alcohols: n-pentanol (NAA), n-
butanol (NBA), and t-butanol (TBA).

In summary the increase in specific conductivity with alcohol addition arises from the increase in the number of charge carriers dissolved in the aqueous phase. The levelling of the conductivity signifies that the liquid crystalline phase boundary has been crossed and that neither the nature of the charge carriers in the aqueous solution nor the viscosity of the aqueous solution vary further with alcohol over the range observed. Although Equation (2) captures the qualitative features of the trends, the equation is not quantitatively obeyed. For example, in the level regions, Equation (2) predicts a conductivity ratio of 10 to 1 for the 0.5 and 0.05 wt % SHBS solutions, whereas the observed ratio is about 5.5 to 1. This disagreement can be explained qualitatively by ionic interactions, but from the results given in Fig. 4 it is more likely that the disagreement has to do with the state of aggregation of alcohol and surfactant in aqueous solution.

NBA and NAA were much more efficient solubilizers of the liquid crystallites than was TBA as indicated by turbidimetry. This finding was reinforced by conductimetric data as shown by Fig. 4 for a 0.5 wt % SHBS dispersion titrated with TBA, NBA, and NAA, respectively. The rise of conductivity to a plateau of different height for each alcohol probably stems from differences in the state of aggregation of the surfactant with alcohol.

Association, and particularly the cooperative association into closed aggregates called micelles, can be probed by conductimetry. Indeed, micelle formation, which represents a sharp change in the state of aggregation of aqueous surfactant, is conventionally determined from conductivity measurements by plotting equivalent conductivity Λ versus $c^{\frac{1}{2}}$, the square root of surfactant concentration (see for example, Mukerjee et al.[15], Mysels and Otter[16]). In the concentration range of incipient micelle formation, the differential conductivity $\frac{d\Lambda}{dc^{\frac{1}{2}}}$ changes sharply because the size of the charge carriers changes. For SDS, a well-known micellizer, Λ versus $c^{\frac{1}{2}}$ changes dramatically upon micelle formation (see Fig. 5a); the micelle aggregation number is about 70-90 and the fraction of bound counterions is about 0.8[17]. Although the charge of the current-carrying micelles is greater than that of monomers or dimers, the large increase in charge carrier size causes $\frac{d\Lambda}{dc^{\frac{1}{2}}}$ to drop sharply. Generally, changes in the current carrier size can be detected by sufficiently sensitive conductivity measurements.

We measured the equivalent conductivity of isotropic SHBS-alcohol systems upon successive dilution with water. Fig. 5b shows Λ versus $c_{SHBS}^{\frac{1}{2}}$ for SHBS-NAA solutions for which NAA/SHBS is 5. All solutions were visually clear over 3 cm pathlengths, apparently scattered no light from the beam of a 3 mW laser, and showed no evidence of birefringence or anisotropy from NMR line width evidence. The slope is everywhere too negative to be fit by the Onsager equation[18], $\Lambda = \Lambda_o - Sc^{\frac{1}{2}}$, which is based on 1:1 unassociated electrolytes and the

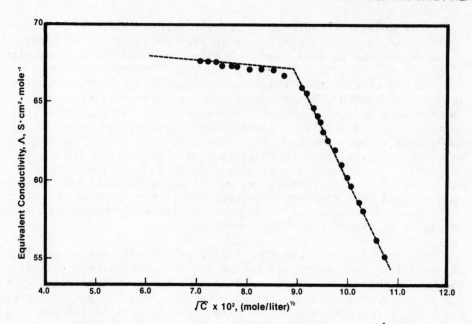

Fig. 5a. Equivalent conductivity ($\Lambda = \dfrac{1000\kappa}{C}$) versus $c^{\frac{1}{2}}$ (moles/litre) for sodium dodecylsulfate (NaLS) in water (from Mysels and Otter 1961

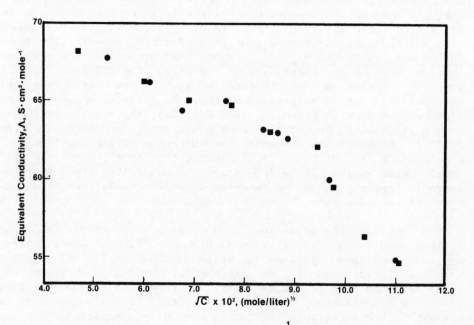

Fig. 5b. Equivalent conductivity versus $c^{\frac{1}{2}}$ for SHBS-NAA-water solution

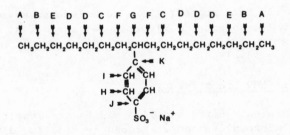

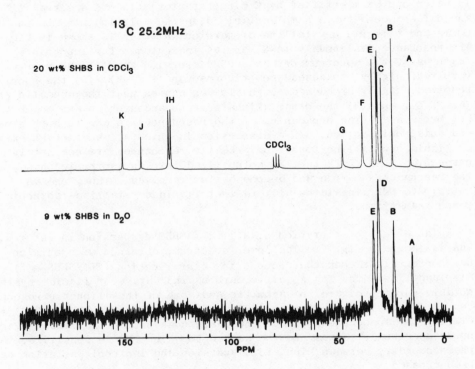

Fig. 6.   ^{13}C NMR spectra of 20 wt % SHBS in CDCl$_3$ and 9 wt % SHBS dispersion in D$_2$O.   At the top are resonance assignments on the structural formula of SHBS.

Debye-Hückel theory. Thus, even at low concentrations of surfactant (c_{SHBS} < 10^{-2} moles/litre), the assumptions implicit in the Onsager equation are no longer valid. However, there is no sharp break in the curve to indicate micelle formation. One possibility is that the alcohol associates enough with the surfactant to reduce the cooperative association of the latter. The result is that small surfactant-alcohol aggregates predominate. An alternative is that the presence of solvating alcohol molecules produces sufficient drag on the charge carriers to alter the differential conductivity. As noted above,

conductimetric data suggest there is molecular association of SHBS
in water in the absence of alcohol. At surfactant concentrations
above the solubility limit, however, alcohol must play a solvating
role.

^{13}C and ^{23}Na NMR Spectroscopy

NMR chemical shifts and line widths are sensitive to molecular
motion and microenvironment. Liquid crystalline dispersions of SHBS
in water can be identified by their characteristic ^{13}C spectra[6,7,19].
The difference between a molecularly disperse solution of SHBS in
$CDCl_3$ and a liquid crystalline dispersion in water is shown in Fig. 6.
The resonance assignments (A-K) are as indicated. The important
features of the spectrum of the SHBS dispersion are (1) the poorly
resolved, highly broadened aromatic resonances (I-K), (2) the poorly
resolved, highly broadened aliphatic resonances near the aromatic ring
(G, F, C), and (3) the other aliphatic resonances which are observable
but broadened. The broadening of the resonances is due to both slow
and anistropic motion. In a dispersion in which all surfactant exists
in liquid crystalline form, the aromatic resonances are completely
unresolved. As surfactant is solubilized into an isotropic phase,
the resonances sharpen and become better resolved. Thus, one may
anticipate NMR linewidths will reflect liquid crystalline-isotropic
phase transitions.

The effect of titration of a 1 wt % SHBS dispersion in water with
TBA is shown in Fig. 7. The lower spectrum, obtained with an alcohol content less than that needed for clarification (TBA/SHBS = 5)
displays linewidths for specific carbons indicative of liquid crystals.
Notably unresolved are the aromatic and some of the aliphatic resonances ($\geq$ 40 ppm). Upon further addition of alcohol (TBA/SHBS = 5.6) to
clarify the suspension, all of the resonances become observable (Fig.
upper spectrum). Hence, to the degree to which NMR is sensitive, the
phase boundary between biphasic dispersion and isotropic solution has
been crossed.

We titrated a 0.5 wt % SHBS dispersion with NAA. Fig. 8 shows
the ^{13}C spectra at NAA/SHBS w/w ratios of 2/1, 3/1, and 4/1, the solutions of which were slightly turbid, translucent, and clear, respectively. The spectrum of the 2/1 dispersion suggests much of the surfactant was in the isotropic phase even though spectroturbidimetric
evidence indicates the system is still biphasic. Although quantitative intensity data from ^{13}C spectra are difficult to obtain, it is
evident from Fig. 8 that the relative height of the C-1 peak, which
corresponds to the C-OH resonance of the alcohol with respect to the
other alcohol resonances is reduced in the liquid crystalline dispersion (bottom) compared to the isotropic solution (top). It is also
obvious that the C-1 line width for the turbid dispersion is greater
than that with higher alcohol content. A likely explanation is that
the alcohol molecules insert themselves into the liquid crystal

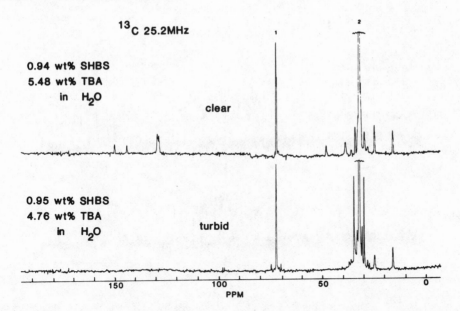

Fig. 7. ^{13}C NMR spectra of a 0.94 wt % SHBS dispersion with different
amounts of TBA added to form turbid (lower) and clear (upper) solutions.
Resonances marked 1 and 2 are from the alcohol with C-1 the C-OH carbon. The remaining resonances are from the surfactant.

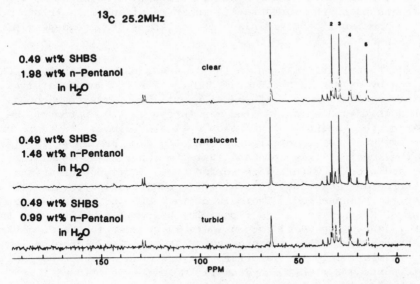

Fig. 8. ^{13}C NMR spectra of a 0.49 wt % SHBS dispersion with various
amounts of n-pentanol added to form turbid (lower), translucent (middle), and clear (upper) solutions. Resonances 1-5 are from n-pentanol
with C-1 the C-OH carbon. The remaining resonances are from the surfactant.

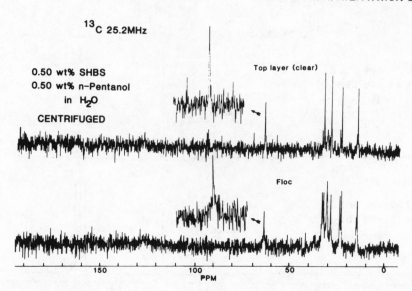

Fig. 9. ^{13}C NMR spectra of a 0.5 wt % SHBS, 0.5 wt % NAA dispersion
which was centrifuged and separated into a floc (lower) and clear
solution (upper). The expanded regions are of the C-1 carbon of the
alcohol.

lamellae, positioning their hydroxylic moieties adjacent to the sulfonate groups of the surfactant. Their resultant anisotropic movement in the lamellae gives rise to the line width broadening of the
C-1 resonances.

Additional information on the interaction of alcohol and SHBS we
obtained by examining a 0.5 wt % SHBS, 0.5 wt % NAA dispersion. This
biphasic system was centrifuged at about 22,000 g's for 3 hours during
which a whitish, semisolid floc was thrown to the bottom of the tube,
rendering the supernatant solution optically clear. ^{13}C spectra
taken of both the top clear phase and the floc are shown in Fig. 9.
From the spectra it is apparent that the supernatant consists of
water and alcohol with little surfactant. It is not clear whether
the surfactant is solubilized at this concentration or the floc was
incompletely separated. The bulk of the SHBS and a considerable
amount of NAA reside in the floc. The hydroxylic C-1 peak of the
alcohol (shown expanded) is considerably broader in the floc than in
the supernatant. The inference again is that the alcohol molecules
align themselves in the lamellar bilayers much as their surfactant
counterparts do, with the hydroxylic moieties positioned in the
water-head group surface zones of the lamellae. At a sufficiently
high concentration of alcohol in the lamellae, the bilayers become
thermodynamically unstable with respect to the isotropic phase. A
similar centrifugation experiment performed on a 0.5 wt % SHBS, 0.5
wt % NBA dispersion in water revealed analogous ^{13}C NMR spectra,

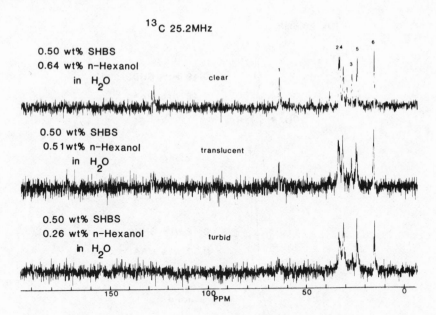

Fig. 10. ^{13}C NMR spectra of a 0.5 wt % SHBS dispersion with various
amounts of n-hexanol added resulting in turbid (lower), translucent
(middle), and biphasic with lower phase clear (upper) solutions.
Resonances 1-6 are from n-hexanol with the C-1 the C-OH carbon.   The
remaining resonances are from the surfactant.

implying a similar mechanism of liquid crystalline dissolution.

    The trend towards enhanced solubilizing power with increasing
lipophilicity, which was found by conductimetry, extends to the almost
water-insoluble alcohol, n-hexanol. Fig. 10 shows the effect of
titration with n-hexanol (NHA) of a 0.5 wt % SHBS dispersion. At NHA/
SHBS w/w ratios of 0.5 and 1, the systems were visually turbid and
translucent dispersions, respectively. At a NHA/SHBS ratio of 1.3,
the suspension had separated to form a clear bottom phase and a thin
layer of opaque liquid on top. The onset of phase separation coincides with the solubility limit of NHA in water. Fig. 10 shows
spectra of the turbid and translucent dispersions as well as the clear
bottom phase at a NHA/SHBS ratio of 1.3. It is quite clear from the
spectra that over this range of alcohol concentrations, the surfactant
passes from the highly anisotropic liquid crystalline phase to a
phase which is quite isotropic. The aromatic resonances are well
resolved in the top spectrum while not observed in the bottom. Even
more striking is the conversion of the hydroxylic C-1 resonance from
a very broad line to a narrow one. Again, the implication is that
the alcohol exists in the liquid crystal much as the surfactant mole-

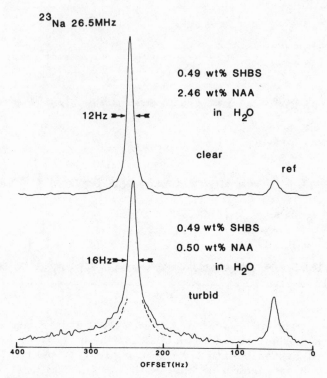

Fig. 11. ^{23}Na NMR spectrum of a 0.5 wt % SHBS dispersion (lower) and a 0.05 wt % SHBS solution (upper) in H_2O.

cules do: its hydroxylic "head" group undergoes slow and anisotropic motion while its aliphatic "tail" group is still moving rapidly and isotropically. Furthermore, n-hexanol is much more efficient at solubilizing the liquid crystals than is NAA, NBA, or TBA. This is to be expected because it is more lipophilic and should partition preferentially into the lamellar phase rather than the aqueous phase.

^{23}Na NMR Spectroscopy

The transition from an isotropic SHBS solution to a biphasic, liquid crystalline dispersion can be readily observed with ^{23}Na NMR also. Shown in Fig. 11 are the ^{23}Na spectra of 0.05 wt % and 0.5 wt % SHBS in water, which are isotropic and biphasic, respectively. The solubility limit of SHBS in water is 0.06 wt % at 25°C[6]. The two noticeable differences in the spectra are in line widths and in chemical shifts. The line width in the dispersion is 3.5 times greater than in the isotropic phase. A change in chemical shift of ca 1 ppm is also observed, with the liquid crystal resonance being

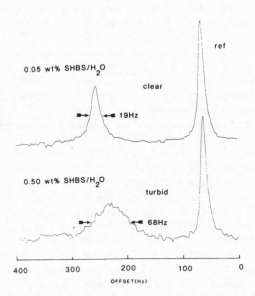

Fig. 12. ^{23}Na NMR spectrum of a 0.49 wt % SHBS dispersion with
various amounts of NAA added resulting in a turbid (lower) and clear
(upper) solution. Dashed line is drawn for a Lorentzian line with
$\Delta \upsilon_{\frac{1}{2}} = 16$ Hz.

more shielded (upfield). This increase in line width and shielding
is consistent with other studies of metal ions in liquid crystals
and micellar solutions and is thought to be due to increased binding
of the sodium ion to the sulfonate head group[20,21].

When NAA is added to a 0.5 wt % SHBS dispersion in water the Na^{+}
resonance narrows and shifts downfield, consistent with the conversion
from liquid crystal to isotropic solution. The comparison between
partially and completely solubilized systems is shown in Fig. 12.   The
turbid dispersion (bottom) has a larger half line-width and the line
shape is not a simple Lorentzian (the dashed line indicates a single
Lorentzian with $\Delta \upsilon_{\frac{1}{2}} = 16$ Hz). The clear isotropic phase has a single
Lorentzian with a narrower line width. Hence, ^{23}Na NMR is also sen-
sitive to liquid crystalline to isotropic phase transitions.

In an attempt to detect any microstructure that might have been
present in the isotropic solution, we made a series of dilutions with
water of a NAA/SHBS w/w ratio of 5/1. There was no evidence within
experimental error of change in either chemical shift or line width

as alcohol concentration varied which might be interpreted as micelle
formation[21]. Thus, either micelles are not present or the effect
of alcohol moderates the Na^+-sulfonate interactions to the extent that
this experiment was insensitive to micelle formation.

Fast-Freeze Transmission Electron Microscopy

In order to visualize directly the effect of alcohol on SHBS
liquid crystalline dispersions, we studied several NAA-SHBS solutions
by fast-freeze, cold-stage electron microscopy[8,9]. Fig. 13a is a
transmission electron micrograph of a hand-shaken dispersion of 0.6
wt % SHBS in water. The round objects in the right-center and lower-
left of the picture are liquid crystalline particles which are embed-
ded in the surrounding ice matrix. Grain boundaries and bend contours
are also visible in the ice. Bend contours are the result of electron
optic contrast mechanisms and are formed by the interaction of the
electron beam with bent or strained areas in an ice crystal. The
appearance of the bend contours alters when Bragg conditions are
changed, the contours moving as the beam divergence is changed or as
the crystal is tilted (Fig. 13b). The bend contours go around the
inclusions, indicating that they are indeed particles contained
within the ice. The round particles are identified as liquid crystals
from the striations inside them, which may be moiré patterns. Like
bend contours, moiré fringes are an electron diffraction effect, which
might be caused by ice crystal planes overlapping an ordered structure
in the frozen liquid crystal. When diffracting conditions are changed
by tilting the sample the appearance of the striations alters (Fig.13b

We also found evidence of liquid crystalline particles in low
weight ratios of dilute aqueous NAA-SHBS solutions. Figs. 14 and 15
are tilt-pairs of micrographs of solutions of 0.418 wt % NAA, 0.697
wt % SHBS and 1.19 wt % NAA, 0.593 wt % SHBS in water systems which
conductimetry and spectroturbidimetry identified as biphasic dispersions. Striations are readily apparent in many of the inclusions,
indicating that they are liquid crystalline in nature. Since some of
the particles have diameters larger than the average sample thickness,
they may have been distorted by the sample preparation procedure.

Unfortunately, from electron microscopy we cannot obtain any
quantitative information about the distribution of particle sizes in
the NAA-SHBS dispersions. This is because 100 keV electrons cannot
penetrate thicker areas of the samples, areas which may contain
larger particles. However, samples of NAA and SHBS in a 2/1 ratio
(Fig. 15) appeared to have a larger proportion of smaller particles
than either 0/1 or 0.6/1 solutions (Figs. 13 and 14).

We have not been able to identify any liquid crystalline particles in solutions of NAA to SHBS ratios greater than 3/1. This is
consistent with other lines of evidence indicating these systems are
indeed isotropic.

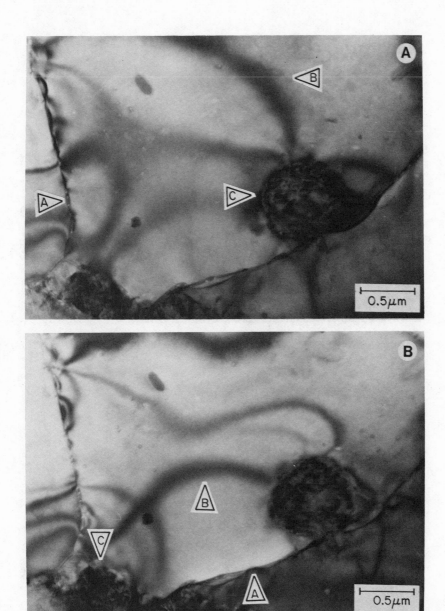

Fig. 13 (a) Electron micrograph of frozen aqueous dispersion of 0.6
wt % SHBS showing grain boundaries (A), bend contours (B), and liquid
crystalline particles containing striations (C). (b) Same area of
sample, but tilted by 1°.

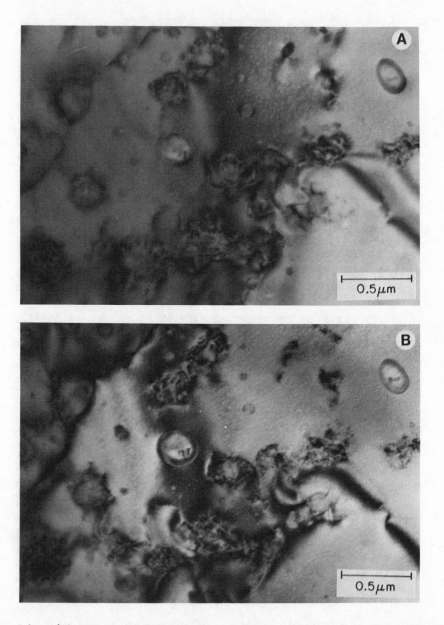

Fig. 14. (a) Electron micrograph of frozen dispersion of 0.418 wt %
n-pentanol (NAA), 0.697 wt % SHBS. (b) Same area of sample, but
tilted by 1°.

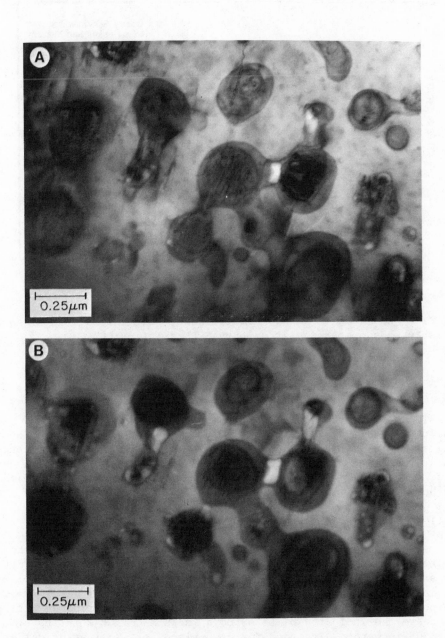

Fig. 15. (a) Electron micrograph of frozen 1.19 wt % n-pentanol, 0.593 wt % SHBS (2:1 ratio) aqueous solution. (b) Same area of sample, but tilted by 1°.

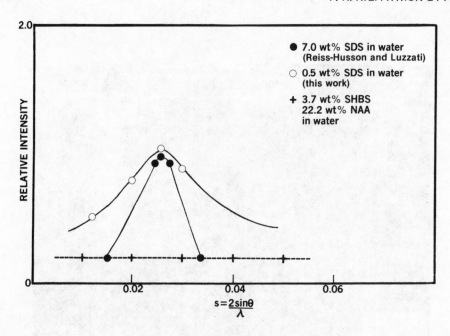

Fig. 16. Small-angle x-ray relative scattering intensities of aqueous
SDS solutions compared with aqueous SHBS solution.

Thus, electron microscopy reveals the existence of liquid crystalline particles in dilute aqueous solutions of NAA and SHBS up to
ratios of at least 2/1. In mixtures containing higher proportions of
alcohol, we saw no structures which we could identify as liquid crystals. Further research will help elucidate the mechanism by which
alcohols solubilize the liquid crystallites.

Small-Angle X-Ray Scattering

In an effort to elucidate any possible microstructure in the
isotropic NAA-SHBS systems, we undertook a small-angle x-ray scattering study. Fig. 16 shows the results for 3.7 wt % SHBS, 22.2 wt %
NAA in water. No appreciable darkening of the Warhaus camera film
was observed for the SHBS solution after an exposure time sufficient
to create the indicated pattern for a known micellar solution of 0.5
wt % SDS in water. Included for comparison is a scattering pattern
created by a 7.0 wt % SDS solution[22]. Similarly, less concentrated
samples of SHBS-NAA isotropic solutions showed no peaks in a plot of
intensity versus scattering vector s. Thus, from small-angle x-ray
scattering we have no evidence of any large aggregate formation in the

clear NAA-SHBS isotropic phase. Of course it is possible that small
aggregates of alcohol-solvated SHBS molecules do exist in solution
but do not provide sufficient electron density contrast to give rise
to scattering peaks.

Effect of NaCl on Aqueous Dispersion

With the exception of NHA, addition of sufficient alcohol to a
biphasic SHBS dispersion yields a clear, isotropic solution. Adding
NHA causes an opaque liquid, rich in alcohol, to appear in the dispersion, before complete liquid crystalline solubilization. This
opaque fluid is apparently a stable SHBS-NHA-water emulsion because it
fails to clear upon centrifugation at about 1000 g's. Addition of
NaCl to the solubilized isotropic systems formed with NBA, TBA, and
NAA causes a phase transformation from which two isotropic phases
result: the bottom phase is largely water and salt with very little
surfactant **or** alcohol while the top phase contains most of the
alcohol and surfactant with a significant amount of water. Fig. 17
shows a series of 0.5 wt % SHBS, 0.5 wt % NaCl in water solutions with
increasing amounts of NAA. At a NAA/SHBS ratio of 4.6/1, the dispersion has separated into two phases, the top one scattering visible
light. Attempts to determine the microstructure of this phase have
revealed only that it weakly scatters x-rays at small values of s.

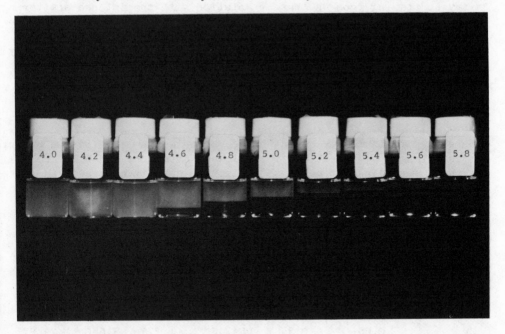

Fig. 17. Titrations of 0.5 wt % SHBS, 0.5 wt % NaCl in water solutions
with increasing amounts of n-pentanol (NAA). Far left solution has NAA/
SHBS (w/w) of 4.0; NAA/SHBS increment from sample to sample is 0.2.

The pattern of phase behaviour seen in mixtures of NaCl, NAA, and SHBS in water is paralleled by mixtures in which the alcohol is NBA or NHA. Above a certain alcohol concentration, the system splits into two fast-settling, apparently isotropic phases; a clear aqueous lower phase and an opalescent surfactant-rich upper phase. From mixing and thermal cycles, both phases appear to be in equilibrium. As the proportion of alcohol is increased, the volume fraction of this upper phase decreases as does the turbidity as illustrated in Fig. 17. The microstructure of the upper phase is still unknown.

Microemulsion Formation

Adding decane 1:1 by volume to mixtures of NaCl-NBA-SHBS that at equilibrium consist of two solution phases yields a microemulsion phase, the appearance of which depends strongly on salt concentration. Table 1 shows the reagent concentrations used. The mixtures at salinities 0.30 and 0.40 split into two phases, the lower of which is surfactant rich, relatively fluid, translucent and is called a microemulsion. At salinities of 0.50 and 0.65, two-phase mixtures resulted with the microemulsion being the upper phase. Our primary tool for characterizing these microemulsions was small-angle x-ray scattering.

Fig. 18 qualitatively compares the relatively low small-angle x-ray scattering from the parent solution with the intense scattering from the microemulsion phase. Thus, the microemulsion formed by the addition of decane to the parent solution possesses considerable microstructure. A size scale can be estimated from the data for any isotropic system from [23]

$$I_{cor} \sim exp \; \frac{-R_G^2 h^2}{3} \qquad \qquad \ldots (3)$$

where I_{cor} is the observed intensity corrected for collimation effects, R_G is a length scale called the radius of gyration, and $h \equiv \frac{4\pi sin\theta}{\lambda}$. If there were disjoint regions of electron density contrast and these

Table 1. Overall Compositions of Components in Microemulsion in Figure 19.

Sample	Initial Salinity	Weight % NaCl	Water	SHBS	NBA	Decane
2	0.30	0.164	54.60	1.777	3.554	39.91
_2_	0.40	0.219	54.56	1.776	3.552	39.90
2̲	0.50	0.274	54.51	1.776	3.552	39.89
2̄	0.65	0.356	54.45	1.775	3.550	39.87

(2̲ denotes a two-phase microemulsion system with the bulk of the surfactant residing in the bottom phase. Similarly 2̄ denotes a two-phase upper microemulsion system.)

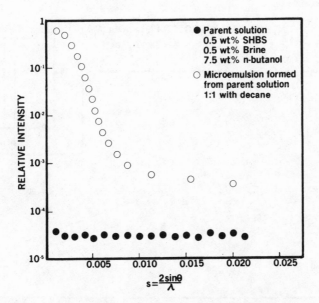

Fig. 18. X-ray scattering relative intensities of microemulsion compared to parent aqueous solution. The data are not corrected for collimation effects.

were more or less convex, R_G would be a measure of their size.   If the regions varied in size, R_G would be an averaged measure of their size. On the other hand, if there are multiply-connected regions of higher and lower electron density contrast — a so-called bicontinuous microstructure[24-29] — R_G would be roughly a measure of their correlation length[29]. Fig. 19 shows the dependence of R_G on salinity as the surfactant-rich microemulsion passes from the bottom phase to the top phase with increasing salinity. The results indicate a coarsening of the microstructure of the microemulsion as the salinity of the transition from lower to upper phase microemulsion is approached. We are presently employing x-ray data such as these, as well as information from other techniques, in order to understand the nature of the microstructure of microemulsion.

Concluding Remarks

    We studied the effect of several low molecular weight alcohols on lamellar liquid crystalline dispersions of the double-tail surfactant SHBS in aqueous solution. At sufficiently high alcohol concentrations, the lamellar phase is solubilized, i.e., it is transformed

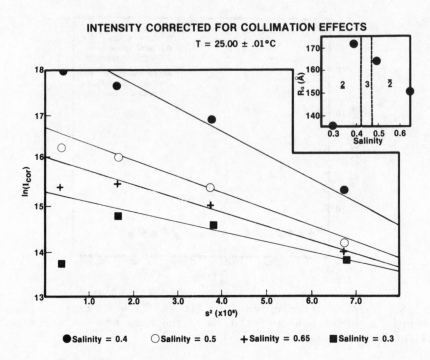

Fig. 19. Effect of salinity on microemulsion radius of gyration, R_G, for SHBS-NBA-decane-brine microemulsions (Compositions presented in Table 1).

into an isotropic phase. The process of solubilization has been studied by a battery of experimental techniques, notably conductimetry ^{13}C and ^{23}Na NMR spectroscopy, small-angle x-ray scattering, and a novel technique for direct visualization of fluid microstructure, fast-freeze cold-stage transmission electron microscopy. Conductimetric evidence indicates there are probably small alcohol-surfactant aggregates in this isotropic phase. Preliminary small-angle x-ray scattering data indicate the aggregates are not as large as SDS micelles, whose diameter is about 40 Å. Conductimetric data indicates no sharp break which could be interpreted as micelle formation.

The process of solubilization of SHBS liquid crystals by alcohols is deduced from ^{13}C NMR evidence. The alcohol molecules partition into the lamellar phase and position themselves in the bilayers with their hydroxylic moieties adjacent to the hydrophilic sulfonate head groups of the surfactant molecules in the surface zones of the lamellae. The alcohol aliphatic "tails" undergo rapid motion as do the surfactant tail groups in the interior of the bilayers. The free energy loss which drives the surfactant from aqueous solution to form

the lamellar phase is probably what drives the alcohol to partition
in the same ordered way in the lamellae. With sufficient alcohol
present, the liquid crystallites become thermodynamically unstable
with respect to the isotropic phase and are solubilized.

The addition of NaCl causes the solubilized isotropic phase to
separate into two isotropic phases: the lower one rich in water and
salt but lean in surfactant and the top one rich in alcohol and surfactant and containing a considerable amount of water. This top
phase scatters light and appears to possess some microstructure. It
is these brine-alcohol-SHBS systems which give rise to microemulsion
upon hydrocarbon addition. The relation between the microstructure
of the oil-free systems and the microstructure of the resulting microemulsion is the object of our ongoing research on microemulsion
structure.

ACKNOWLEDGEMENTS

This research was supported by the National Institutes of Health
and the Department of Energy. The authors wish to thank K. E. Bennett,
and W. R. Rossen for helpful suggestions and information.
One of us (E. W. K.) would like to thank R. W. Hendricks, J. S. Lin,
and R. Triolo of Oak Ridge National Laboratory for their help in
designing the modified Kratky camera.

REFERENCES

1. R. J. M. Tausk, J. Karmiggelt, C. Oudshoorn, and J. Th. G. Over-
    beck, Biophys. Chem., 1, 175 (1974).
2. J. E. Puig, H. T. Davis, L. E. Scriven, and W. G. Miller, 1981,
    to be presented at 90th AIChE National Meeting, Houston, Texas,
    April 5-9, 1981.
3. S. Friberg, I. Buraczewska, and J. C. Ruvey in "Micellization,
    Solubilization, and Microemulsions", Vol. 2, K. L. Mittal, Ed.,
    Plenum Press, New York, 1977, p. 901.
4. P. K. Kilpatrick, C. A. Gorman, H. T. Davis, W. G. Miller, and
    L. E. Scriven, manuscript in preparation.
5. S. Friberg, P. O. Jansson, and E. Cederberg, J. Coll.and Inter.
    Sci., 55, 614 (1976).
6. E. I. Franses, H. T. Davis, W. G. Miller, and L. E. Scriven,
    Paper presented in the symposium on Chemistry of Oil Recovery
    at the 175th National Meeting of the American Chemical Society,
    Anaheim, Calif., March 13, 1978; ACS Symp. Ser. 1979
7. E. I. Franses, Ph.D. Thesis, University of Minnesota, June 1979.
8. Y. Talmon, H. T. Davis, L. E. Scriven, and E. L. Thomas, Rev.
    Sci. Instr., 50, 698 (1979).
9. Y. Talmon, Ph.D. Thesis, University of Minnesota, March 1979.
10. T. P. Russell, R. S. Stein, M. K. Kopp, R. E. Zedler, R. W. Hen-
    dricks, and J. S. Lin, 1979, ORNL-TM# 6678, Oak Ridge National
    Laboratory, Oak Ridge, Tennessee, 37830.

11. P. W. Schmidt, Acta Cryst., 19, 938 (1965).
12. L. Magid, U.S. Dept. of Energy Quarterly Report on Chemicals for Enhanced Oil Recovery, Oak Ridge National Laboratory, Oak Ridge, Tennessee, 37830, July 1980, p.23.
13. W. J. Benton and D. F. Evans, 1980, unpublished results.
14. J. E. Puig, H. T. Davis, W. G. Miller, and L. E. Scriven, 1980, unpublished results.
15. P. Mukerjee, K. J. Mysels, and C. I. Dulin, J. Physic. Chem., 62 1390 (1958).
16. K. J. Mysels and R. J. Otter, J. Colloid Sci., 16, 474 (1961).
17. C. Botre, V. L. Crescenzi, and A. Mele, J. Physic, Chem., 63, 650 (1959).
18. L. Onsager, Physik Z., 27, 388 (1926).
19. E. I. Franses, J. F. Puig, Y. Talmon, W. G. Miller, L. E. Scriven, and H. T. Davis, J. Physic. Chem., 84, 1547 (1980).
20. H. Gustavsson and B. Lindman, J. Amer. Chem. Soc., 97, 3923 (1975).
21. H. Gustavsson and B. Lindman, J. Amer. Chem. Soc., 100, 4547 (1978).
22. F. Reiss-Husson and V. Luzzati, J. Physic. Chem. 68, 3504 (1964).
23. A. Guinier and G. Fournet, "Small-Angle Scattering of X-Rays", John Wiley and Sons, New York, 1955, Chapter 2.
24. L. E. Scriven, Nature, 263, 123 (1976) and in "Micellization, Solubilization, and Microemulsions", Vol. 2, K. L. Mittal, Ed., Plenum Press, New York, 1977, p. 877.
25. J. C. Hatfield, Ph.D. Thesis, University of Minnesota, March 1978.
26. M. Lagues, R. Ober, and C. Taupin, J. Physique Lett., 39, L-487 (1978).
27. B. Lindman, N. Kamenka, T. M. Kathopoulis, B. Brun, and P. G. Nilsson, J. Physic. Chem., 84, 2485 (1980).
28. K. E. Bennett, J. C. Hatfield, H. T. Davis, C. W. Macosko, and L. E. Scriven, paper presented at the Industrial Sub-Committee of the Faraday Division of the Chemical Society's meeting on "The Physical Chemistry of Microemulsions", Sept. 15-16, 1980.
29. E. W. Kaler and S. Prager, presented at the 5th International Small-Angle Scattering Conference, Berlin, West Germany, Oct. 6-10, 1980, manuscript in preparation.

DISCUSSION

Prof. B. Lindman: You make very adequate use of NMR to distinguish between different phases present. One could perhaps comment that the line broadening (in ^1H or ^{13}C NMR) is connected to large aggregates and not to liquid crystals as opposed to isotropic solutions. Therefore, rod micelles and large vesicles give broad signals while cubic liquid crystals give narrow lines.

Prof. H. T. Davis: We have previously determined ^{13}C NMR spectra of the SHBS surfactant in the bulk smectic phase (ref. 6), in small

vesicles (E. I. Franses, Y. Talmon, L. E. Scriven, H. T. Davis, and
W. G. Miller, J. Colloid and Interface Sci., submitted), and in
liposomes (F. D. Blum and W. G. Miller, J. Colloid and Interface Sci.,
to be submitted; E. I. Franses, K. Rose, F. D. Blum, P. S. Russo,
R. G. Bryant, and W. G. Miller, J. Colloid and Interface Sci., to be
submitted) as well as of SDS in spherical and in presumably metastable
rod micelles (E. I. Franses, H. T. Davis, W. G. Miller, and L. E.
Scriven, J. Physic. Chem., 84, 2413. (1980)). On the basis of these
studies, we feel the transition observed is from the smectic phase
to an isotropic phase in which there may be appreciable molecular
association.

Dr W. J. Benton: First I would like to concur with your results on
the lamellar →isotropic phase transition. We have also seen this
in Texas 1-brine-n-propanol, but in some of the commercial systems we
have also observed a lamellar → lamellar/cubic → cubic →cubic/iso-
tropic transition. Have you observed such a transition in the Texas
1-brine-higher alcohols systems?

Prof. H. T. Davis: In all of the SHBS systems we studied in the
absence of NaCl the lamellar to isotropic phase transition was the
only phase transition observed. In the presence of NaCl, the systems
split into two fast-separating isotropic phases before this transition
occurred. The upper phase in these brine systems must have considerable microstructure to judge from the turbidity we saw, but we have
found no evidence of a cubic phase.

Prof. F. Franks: (1) Are there ice crystals in the samples photo-
graphed by EM? The egg-shaped structures can be associated with them.
(2) Any experimental technique that involves freezing however fast,
is likely to produce artifacts arising from marked concentration
changes in the system during the crystallisation of ice in the aqueous
phase. The only way to avoid phase separation during cooling is to
vitrify the system, for purposes of electron microscopy. I doubt
whether the very high cooling rates required for vitrification can be
achieved with systems that have a low viscosity and a relatively high
water content.

Prof. H. T. Davis: Indeed, with the double-film technique, we are
not able to vitrify aqueous systems. The size of the grains of ice
in Figures 13, 14 and 15 indicates that the cooling rate is much
lower than that required to capture water in an amorphous state. Even
so, for structures requiring long times to nucleate and grow, for
example, liquid crystals and vesicles (ref. 9) and perhaps even micelles, molecular rearrangement during phase separation can be avoided.
From the supporting evidence of spectroturbidimetry, conductimetry,
and NMR, this seems likely for the dispersed liquid crystalline phase
of low alcohol content. In systems with higher proportions of alcohol,
however, fast-freezing may induce appreciable transport during phase
transformation. We have chosen not to publish micrographs of these

systems (to which your question regarding the egg structures is
directed) until we are able to interpret fully the observed structures.

CONNECTION BETWEEN CHEMICAL RATE COEFFICIENTS AND TWO-PARTICLE

CORRELATION FUNCTIONS IN AGGREGATED SYSTEMS

Sz. Vass

Chemistry Department
Central Research Institute for Physics of the Hungarian
Academy of Sciences
H-1525 Budapest, P.O. Box 49

INTRODUCTION

The present paper deals with some aspects of chemical rate
coefficients in the liquid phase in the case when reactants are incorporated into more or less stable and closed aggregates of surface
active molecules. The term aggregate covers here a wide range of
theoretically different formations from micelles to microemulsions.

An ever increasing attention has been paid in the last decade to
investigations of rate coefficients and reaction mechanisms in the
presence of microaggregates[1-21]. The exact treatment of these
reactions is very difficult for two reasons. First, the processes
involved in aggregate formation[22-35] and in particle incorpora-
tion[36-39] are extremely complicated. Second, the systems under
consideration are so small[24,29-32] that the use of concepts of
classical statistical physics elaborated for large systems e.g. diffusion[15,18,19] can be questioned. Thus, it seems that in the case of
microaggregates the classical concepts need a careful reformula-
tion[40-41].

Experimental evidence[13,14] suggests that random collision
models[3,13,20,21,42] are adequate to describe chemical kinetics in
these systems. Our aim is to express the co-efficients of random
collision models using the concepts of liquid physics and to discuss
some features of the coefficients.

GENERAL CONSIDERATIONS

In order to describe observable phenomena due to chemical reactions in microaggregates, the first step is to determine the processes occurring in individual microaggregates. The chemical reaction is taken to be a result of reactive collisions between chaotically moving particles and the rate coefficients correspond to collision densities[42,43] which are calculated from the average number of reactive collisions per unit time.

In order to simplify the very complicated calculations[44] the following assumptions are made:

a. The processes are restricted to irreversible bimolecular reactions of type $A + B \longrightarrow C$.

b. Reactant molecules of type A and B are taken to be hard-core spheres with radii r_A and r_B, respectively. The interaction between two reactant molecules depends only on their distance from each other, described e.g. either by hard-core or by Lennard-Jones potentials and the spatial distribution of molecules is not affected by their internal degrees of freedom.

c. Colliding molecules combine a reaction product molecule with probability p_r which is supposed to be independent of the collision probability.

d. The system is in equilibrium; this state is not perturbed by chemical reactions.

The Hamiltonian has the form:

$$H(q_1 \ldots q_M, p_1 \ldots p_M, Q_1 \ldots Q_N, P_1 \ldots P_N) = \sum_i^M \frac{p_i^2}{2m_i} + \sum_j^N \frac{P_j^2}{2m_j} +$$

$$+ V(q_1 \ldots q_M, Q_1 \ldots Q_N)$$

where (q,p) are space coordinates and momenta of the reactants, (Q,P) are generalized space coordinates and momenta of all other molecules. The interaction potential is divided into three parts as

$$V(q_1 \ldots q_M, Q_1 \ldots Q_N) = \sum_{i \le i < j \le M} \phi_1(|q_i - q_j|) + \sum_i \sum_j \phi_2(q_i, Q_j) + \sum_{i \le i < j \le N} \phi_3(Q_i, Q_j) \quad ..(2.2)$$

The first term of the potential function describes the interaction between reactants (see condition b.), the second term stands for the interaction between the reactants and the other (among them the aggregate) molecules. The last term takes into account the effect of the structure of the liquid.

Note that M and N are the numbers of reactant and of other molecules, respectively, the quantities q,p,Q,P are vectors and the integration with respect to dq,dp,dQ,dP denotes a threefold integration.

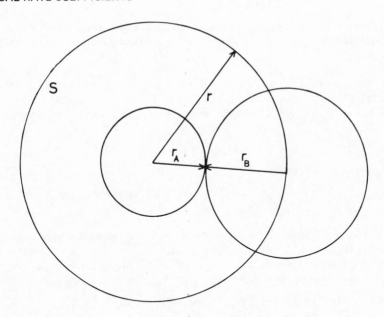

Fig.1a.   Definition of the collision boundary for hard-core spheres.

AVERAGE NUMBER OF COLLISIONS PER UNIT TIME

        In order to evaluate the average number of collisions per unit
time, one has first to determine the geometrical condition of collision for a chosen pair of reactants. Let us introduce the concept
of collision boundary S_{ij} for particles with convex boundaries i,j as
follows: let the particle j of type B move around the fixed particle
i of type A in such a way that their relative orientation remains
unchanged and that their surfaces remain in contact. The collision
boundary S_{ij} is defined as the set of points representing all possible
geometrical positions which can be taken by the centre of mass point
of particle j.

        In the simple case of hard-core spheres of radii r_A and r_B the
collision boundary is a spherical surface of radius $r = r_A + r_B$ which
is well known from the textbooks of statistical physics and physical
chemistry; see Fig 1a.

        Let $\Delta q_{ij} = (p_j - p_i)\Delta t$ be the relative displacement vector of
particles i,j during Δt and let us define the volume element $\Delta\omega_{ij}$ by
the integral:

$$\Delta\omega_{ij} = - \int_{\tilde{S}_U} (\mathbf{n}\Delta q_{ij})dS = - \Delta t \int_{\tilde{S}_U} (p_j - p_i) \frac{\text{grad } S_{ij}}{|\text{grad } S_{ij}|} dS \qquad \ldots(3.1)$$

where $\mathbf{n}$ is the unit normal vector of S_{ij} in the surface element dS and the integration has to be carried out over that region of the collision boundary where we have for the inner product the inequality $(|\Delta q_{ij}) < 0$.

If and only if the centre of mass point of particle j falls into the volume element $\Delta\omega_{ij}$, will particle j impinge on particle i during Δt, see Fig. 1b. This event is represented by the characteristic function

$$f_{ij} = f_{ij} \ (\Delta t, q_i, q_j, p_i, p_j) \ = \ \begin{cases} 1, \text{ if } q_j \ \epsilon\Delta\omega_{ij} \\ \\ 0, \text{ otherwise} \end{cases} \qquad \ldots(3.2)$$

Since a collision of two particles is a mutual event, the characteristic function of their collision ψ_{ij} has to be a symmetric function in the indices; this condition is satisfied if it is expressed as the arithmetic mean of f_{ij} and f_{ji} in the form

$$\psi_{ij} = \frac{1}{2} \ (f_{ij} + f_{ji}) \ = \ \begin{cases} 1, \text{ if } q_j\epsilon\Delta\omega_{ij} \text{ and } q_i\epsilon\Delta\omega_{ji} \\ \\ 0, \text{ otherwise} \end{cases} \qquad \ldots(3.3)$$

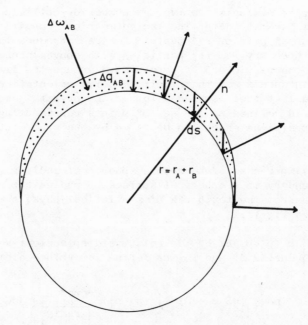

Fig. 1b. Determination of the volume element $\Delta\omega_{ij}$ by the collision boundary and by the relative displacement of moving hard-core spheres.

The total number of collisions between reactants of type A and B observed in Δt is a random function of the reactant coordinates and momenta and it is given by the summation of the characteristic functions of two-particle collisions as

$$\psi(\Delta t) = \psi(\Delta t_1 q_1 \ldots q_{m1} \; p_1 \ldots p_M)$$

$$= \sum_i^{N_A} \sum_j^{N_B} \psi_{ij}(\Delta t, q_i, q_j, p_i, p_j) + o(\Delta t) \qquad \ldots(3,4)$$

N_A and N_B are the numbers of the A and B type reactants involved, $N_A + N_B = M$, $o(\Delta t)$ describes the number of ternary, quaternary etc. collisions. The average number of collisions $\mu(\Delta t)$ is given as

$$\mu(\Delta t) = \int \psi(\Delta t, q_1 \ldots q_M, \; p_1 \ldots p_M) dW \; (q_1 \ldots q_M, \; p_1 \ldots p_M) \qquad \ldots(3.5)$$

where dW is the statistical weight of finding the reactants around coordinates and momenta $q_1 \ldots q_M$, $p_1 \ldots p_M$ and the other particles around generalized coordinates and generalized momenta $Q_1 \ldots Q_N$, $P_1 \ldots P_N$. For equilibrium systems the statistical weight dW is given by the Gibbs distribution function

$$dW = Z^{-1} \exp\left[-\frac{1}{kT} \left(\sum_i^M \frac{p_i^2}{2m_i} + \sum_j^N \frac{P_j^2}{2m_j} + V(q_1 \ldots q_M, Q_1 \ldots Q_N) \right) \right] d\Gamma \quad \ldots(3.6)$$

In Eq. (3.6) Z is the system integral, k is the Boltzmann-constant, T is the absolute temperature and $d\Gamma$ is the volume element of the phase space. Substituting this formula into Eq. (3.5) and integrating with respect the variables $Q_1 \ldots Q_N$, $P_1 \ldots P_N$ which have no direct effect on the integrand, Eq. (3.5) transforms to

$$\mu(\Delta t) = CV^{-M} \int \psi(\Delta t, \; q_1 \ldots q_M, \; p_1 \ldots p_M) \exp\left[-\frac{1}{kT} \sum_i^M \frac{p_i^2}{2m_i} \right] \times$$

$$\times F_M \; (q_1 \ldots q_M) \; dp_1 \ldots dp_M \; dq_1 \ldots dq_M \qquad \ldots(3.7)$$

where C is a constant, V is the volume of the system, $F_M(q_1 \ldots q_M)$ is the M-particle correlation function derived from the interaction part of the Hamiltonian in Eq. (2.2) for details see (45-47) in the form

$$F_M(q_1 \ldots q_M) =$$

$$= V^M \exp\left[-\frac{1}{kT} \sum_{1 \leq i < j \leq M} \phi_1(|q_i - q_j|)\right] \cdot \int \exp\left[-\frac{1}{kT} \sum_i^M \sum_j^N \phi_2(q_i, Q_j)\right]$$

$$\sum_{1 \leq i < j \leq N} \phi_3(Q_i, Q_j)\right] dQ_1 \ldots dQ_N$$

$$= V^M \phi_0(q_1 \ldots q_M) \exp\left[-\frac{1}{kT} \sum_{1 \leq i < j \leq M} \phi_A(|q_i - q_j|)\right] \qquad \ldots(3.8)$$

Since $\psi(\Delta t)$ is a sum of characteristic functions depending on two-particle coordinates and $F_M(q_1 \ldots q_M)$ is a symmetrical function of its arguments, $\mu(\Delta t)$ can be expressed by an integral of the two-particle correlation function $F_2(q_1, q_2)$, (see (45-47) as

$$\mu(\Delta t) = CV^{-M} \int \sum_i^{N_A} \sum_j^{N_B} \psi_{ij}(\Delta t, q_i, q_j, p_i, p_j) F_M(q_1 \ldots q_M)$$

$$\exp\left[-\frac{1}{kT} \sum_e^M \frac{p_e^2}{2m_e}\right] \times dp_1 \ldots dp_M dq_1 \ldots dq_M$$

$$= CV^{-M} \sum_i^{N_A} \sum_j^{N_B} \int \psi_{ij}(\Delta t, q_i, q_j, p_i, p_j) F_M(q_1 \ldots q_M) \exp\left[-\frac{1}{kT} \sum_e^M \frac{p_e^2}{2m_e}\right] \times$$

$$\times dp_1 \ldots dp_M dq_1 \ldots dq_M$$

$$= CV^{-2} N_A N_B \int \psi_{AB}(\Delta t, q_A, q_B, p_A, p_B) F_2(q_A, q_B) \exp\left[-\frac{1}{2kT}\left(\frac{p_A^2}{m_A} + \frac{p_B^2}{m_B}\right)\right] \times$$

$$\times dp_A dp_B dq_A dq_B \qquad \ldots(3.9)$$

In the last line of Eq.
coordinates of different type reactants. The two-particle correlation function $F_2(q_1, q_2)$ can be reduced to the product of a one-particle function $F_1(q_1)$ and a conditional two-particle function $F_2(q_2/q_1)^{(45-47)}$ of the form

$$F_2(q_2, q_1) = F_1(q_1) F_2(q_2/q_1) \qquad \ldots(3.10)$$

Substituting Eq. (3.10) into Eq. (3.9) and taking into consideration that the characteristic function ψ_{AB} is non zero only in the region $\Delta\omega_{AB}$ where it is equal to 1, the final form to be discussed in the following is obtained as

$$\mu(\Delta t) = C \frac{N_A N_B}{V} \cdot \int \frac{F_1(q_A)}{V} dq_A \int F_2(q_B/q_A)dq_B \exp\left[-\frac{1}{2kT}(\frac{P_A^2}{m_A} + \frac{P_B^2}{m_B})\right]$$

$$dp_A dp_B \quad \Delta\omega_{AB}(q_A, p_A, p_B) \qquad\qquad ...(3.11)$$

RATE COEFFICIENTS IN DIFFERENT MEDIA

Until this point, our considerations apply to arbitrary gas and condensed phase systems. In Eq. (3.8) function ϕ_0 contains the boundary information for reactants: in gases and liquids, where no aggregates are present, ϕ_0 is non-zero for the entire reaction vessel and V is equal to its volume. In this case F_1 is constant and in isotropic medium $F_2(q_2/q_1)$ is a function of the coordinate differences (45-47), thus

$$F_1(q_1) \quad = 1$$

$$F_2(q_2/q_1) = g(|q_2-q_1|) = g(q) \qquad\qquad ...(4.1)$$

where $g(q)$ is the so called pair-correlation function. The integration in Eq. (3.11) in this case reduces to a simple integration over the collision boundary; using spherical polar-coordinates on the collision boundary S_{AB} the inner integral in Eq. (3.11) leads to the simple expression

$$\int_{\Delta\omega_{AB}} F_2(q_B/q_A)dq_B = \Delta t\left| p_{AB}\right| \int_0^{2\pi} \int_0^{\pi/2} v^2 g(r) \sin\delta\cos\delta d\delta d\phi = r^2\pi g(r)\left| p_{AB}\right| \Delta t$$

$$...(4.2)$$

and $g(r)$ is the value of the pair-correlation function at the collision boundary S_{AB}. Hence, integrating with respect to q_A and over the momentum space, and finally, taking into account that the average number of reactive collisions in Δt corresponds to the increase $N_r = \lambda N_A N_B \Delta t$ in reaction product molecules, from comparison of this formula and of the result of the integration the rate coefficient λ is given as

$$\lambda = \frac{r^2 \pi g(r)}{V} \, p_r C \int \left| p_{AB} \right| \, \exp \left[-\frac{1}{2kT} \left(\frac{P_A^2}{m_A} + \frac{P_B^2}{m_B} \right) \right] dp_A dp_B$$

$$= \frac{r^2 \pi g(r)}{V} \, p_r C \overline{p}_{AB}(T) \qquad\qquad\qquad \ldots (4.3)$$

Some features of bimolecular rate coefficients are apparent from Eq. (4.3). The rate coefficient Λ is inversely proportional to the volume of the reaction vessel and it shows Maxwellian-type temperature dependence in $C\overline{p}_{AB}(T)$. The factor $r^2 \pi g(r)$ shows the effect of reactant size and of solution structure, p_r is defined in Section 2, in condition c. If the pair-correlation function is expressed in terms of particle density i.e. as a virial series,[45] in the case of hard-core potentials for very dilute systems Eq. (4.3) reproduces the classical expression for gas phase rate coefficients[48].

In the case of aggregate formation, the function in Eq. (3.8) is supposed to differ from zero in the finite volume of the aggregate V_{Ag}; the basic assumptions listed in Section 2 are completed with this condition. The evaluation of Eq. (3.11) is not a simple task and therefore we restrict ourselves to its qualitative discussion.

According to theoretical considerations and to experimental evidence[49,50] an aggregate is characterized by rapidly varying forces in the neighbourhood of its boundary; because of its small size the boundary effect cannot be neglected and thus it cannot be considered isotropic[45-47,49,50]. As a consequence of this fact, F_1 is not a constant function inside the microaggregate and the conditional two-particle correlation function cannot be replaced by the pair-correlation function $g(r)$. Instead of $g(r)$ the form $F_2 = F_2(r, \delta, \phi, \delta_0, \phi_0 q_A)$ has to be used which generally depends on the orientation of q_A and the relative momentum p_{AB} (see Fig. 2). The inner integral in Eq. (3.11) can be written as

$$\int_{\Delta\omega_{AB}} F_2(q_B/q_A) dq_B = \left| p_{AB} \right| \Delta t \int_0^{2\pi} \int_0^{\pi/2} F_2(r,\delta,\phi,\delta_0,\phi_0 \, q_A) r^2 \cos\delta \sin\delta \, d\delta \, d\phi$$

$$\ldots (4.4)$$

and, in order to express the rate coefficient λ_{Ag} it has to be averaged over the possible orientations of q_A and p_{AB} as

$$\lambda_{Ag} = \frac{r^2}{V_{Ag}} \, p_r \, C \, \overline{p}_{AB}(T) \int \frac{F_1(q_A)}{V_{Ag}} dq_A \, \times$$

$$\times \int_0^{2\pi} \int_0^{\pi/2} \sin\delta_0 \, d\delta_0 \, d\phi_0 \int_0^{2\pi} \int_0^{\pi/2} F_2(r,\delta,\phi,\delta_0,\phi_0 \, q_A) \cos\,\delta . \sin\delta . d\delta d\phi \quad \ldots (4.5)$$

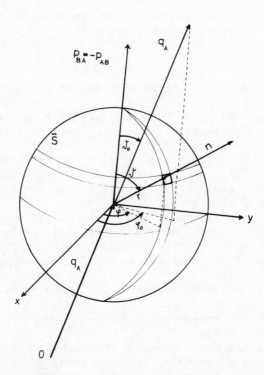

Fig.2. Spherical polar coordinate system connected to the relative momentum vector of the colliding hard-core spheres for the calculation of rate coefficients.

The explicit temperature dependence of the rate coefficient is of the same form, as in the case of isotropic solutions cf. Eq. (4.3). The rate coefficient is inversely proportional to the aggregate volume V_{Ag}; if the size distribution of microaggregates is not so narrow as it is usually supposed, its effect on the reaction kinetics cannot be neglected.

The integrals in Eq. (4.5) define an average spatial correlation which can strongly depend on the type of aggregating molecules and of reactants. If reactants are found in the boundary region of the microaggregate, the effect of the fields on the reaction probability p_r has to be taken into account. These effects - which I cannot discuss in detail at the present level of my knowledge - can result in a further deviation of λ_{Ag} from the rate coefficient determined in isotropic solutions.

ACKNOWLEDGEMENT

The author is indebted to Dr G. Jancso and to Dr R Schiller from the Central Research Institute for Physics, and to Dr G. Putirskaya

from the Central Research Institute for Chemistry of the Hungarian
Academy of Sciences for valuable discussions.

REFERENCES

1. E. H. Cordes (ed.): Reaction Kinetics in Micelles. Plenum Press,
    New York, 1973.
2. J. H. Fendler and E. J. Fendler: Catalysis in Micellar and
    Macromolecular Systems. Academic Press, New York, 1975.
3. M. Tachiya, Chem. Phys. Letters 33, 289 (1975).
4. K. Martinek, A. K. Yatsimirski, A. V. Levashov and I. V. Berezin,
    in: Micellization, Solubilization and Microemulsions, ed. by
    K. L. Mittal, vol. 2, 489. Plenum Press, New York, (1977).
5. L. S. Romsted, ibid., vol. 2, 509.
6. M. Wong and J. K. Thomas, ibid., vol. 2, 647.
7. R. A. Mackay, K. Letts and C. Jones, ibid., vol. 2, 801.
8. Y. -C. Jean and H. J. Ache, J. Am. Chem. Soc. 99, 7504 (1977).
9. J. K. Thomas, F. Grieser and M. Wong, Ber. Bunsenges. Phys.
    Chem. 82, 937 (1978)
10. L. K. Patterson and K. Hasegawa, Ber. Bunsenges. Phys. Chem.
    82, 951 (1978).
11. A. Henglein, Th. Proske and W. Schnecke, Ber. Bunsenges. Phys.
    Chem. 82, 956, (1978).
12. E. D. Handel and H. J. Ache, J. Chem. Phys. 71, 2083 (1979).
13. P. Infelta and M. Grätzel, J. Chem. Phys. 70, 179 (1979).
14. G. Rothenberger, P. Infelta and M. Grätzel, J. Phys. Chem. 83,
    1871 (1979).
15. U. Gösele, U.K.A. Klein and M. Hauser, Chem. Phys. Letters 68,
    291 (1979).
16. S. J. Gregoritch and J. K. Thomas, J. Phys. Chem. 84, 1491 (1980)
17. C. A. Jones, L. E. Weaner and R. A. Mackay, J. Phys. Chem. 84,
    1495 (1980).
18. M. Tachiya, Chem. Phys. Letters 69, 605 (1980).
19. M. D. Hatlee, J. J. Kozak, G. Rothenberger, P. Infelta and
    M. Grätzel, J. Phys. Chem. 84, 1508 (1980).
20. Sz. Vass, Chem. Phys. Letters 70, 135 (1980).
21. M. D. Hatlee and J. J. Kozak, J. Chem. Phys. 72, 4358 (1980).
22. I. Langmuir, J. Chem. Phys. 6, 873 (1938).
23. C. Tanford: The Hydrophobic Effect. John Wiley, New York, (1973).
24. J. N. Israelachvili, D. J. Mitchell and B. W. Ninham, J. Chem.
    Soc. Farad. Trans. II. 72, 1525 (1975).
25. C. Tanford, in: Micellization, Solubilization and Microemulsions,
    ed. by K. L. Mittal, vol. 1, 119. Plenum Press, New York, (1977)
26. K. S. Birdi, ibid., vol. 1, 151.
27. H. F. Eicke, ibid., vol. 1, 429.
28. A. S. Kertes, ibid., vol. 1, 445.
29. P. Mukerjee, ibid., vol. 1, 171.
30. E. Ruckenstein, ibid. vol. 2, 755.
31. J. Th. G. Overbeek, in: Faraday Discussions No. 65, 7 (1978).
32. E. A. G. Aniansson, Ber. Bunsenges. Phys. Chem. 82, 981 (1978).

33. H. Hoffmann, Ber. Bunsenges. Phys. Chem. 82, 989 (1978).
34. K. S. Birdi, H. N. Singh and S. U. Dalsager, J. Phys. Chem. 83, 2733 (1979).
35. C. -U. Herrmann and M. Kahlweit, J. Phys. Chem. 84, 1536 (1980).
36. A. Kitahara and K. Kon-no, in: Micellization, Solubilization and Microemulsions, ed. by K. L. Mittal, vol. 2, 675. Plenum Press, New York, (1977).
37. M. Aikawa, A. Yekta and N. J. Turro, Chem. Phys. Letters 68, 285 (1979).
38. Y. -C. Jean, B. Djermouni and H. J. Ache, in: Solution Chemistry of Surfactants, ed. by K. L. Mittal, vol. 1, 129.
39. P. Mukerjee, A. V. Sapre and J. P. Mittal, Chem. Phys. Letters 69, 121 (1980).
40. T. L. Hill: Thermodynamics of Small Systems. Benjamin, New York, (1963).
41. L. R. Fisher and D. G. Oakenfull, Chem. Soc. Rev. 6, 25 (1977).
42. D. A. McQuerrie, J. Chem. Phys. 38, 433 (1963).
43. D. T. Gillespie, J. Stat. Phys. 16, 311 (1977).
44. Sz. Vass, to be published.
45. I. Z. Fisher: Statistical Theory of Liquids. The University of Chicago Press, Chicago, 1964.
46. H. N. V. Temperley, J. S. Rowlinson and G. S. Rushbroke: Physics of Simple Liquids. North Holland, Amsterdam, 1968.
47. N. N. Bogoljubov: Selected Papers, vol. 2. Naukova Dumka, Kiev, (1970) (in Russian).
48. K. J. Laidler: Theories of Chemical Reaction Rates, McGraw Hill, New York, (1969).
49. J. N. Israelachvili, in: Faraday Discussions No. 65, 20 (1978).
50. B. W. Ninham, J. Phys. Chem. 84, 1423 (1980).

DISCUSSION

Dr J. F. Holzwarth: The stochastic theory and the theory of the activated state (Eyring) yield the same results if one works under the condition of large numbers of reactants. Under which experimental conditions do you expect different results from these two theories?

Dr S. Vass: I do not expect any deviation from these theories. In the averaging procedure used in my calculations a large sub-system of micro-aggregates is tacitly supposed with microaggregates containing the given (small) number of reactants. This type of averaging results in a formula containing the two-particle correlation function; this function is characteristic of the state of the medium (dilute gas, dense gas or liquid) in which the reaction takes place.

However, a further evaluation of experimental data is needed to verify the correctness of this formula.

Prof. H. T. Davis: You state that your singlet distribution function is not constant when the fluid contains aggregates even though the

fluid is isotropic. Does this not mean that you define the singlet
distribution function without respect to a coordinate system fixed in
an aggregate? If so, the situation is similar in molecular fluids.
If one defines the singlet density of the fluid relative to a given
molecule, this so-defined density is the pair correlation function
times the bulk phase density.

Dr S. Vass: We have to distinguish between isotropic fluid and
interior of an aggregate. Rigorously, the singlet distribution function is constant in an infinite isotropic liquid or gas. However,
the singlet distribution function is not constant in the vicinity of
walls even in the before-mentioned media. Inside a microaggregate
the reactants are close to the aggregate surface and considering this
case I have no reason for supposing a constant one particle (i.e.
singlet) distribution function.

FAST DYNAMIC PROCESSES IN THE HYDROCARBON TAIL REGION OF

PHOSPHOLIPID BILAYERS

J. F. Holzwarth, W. Frisch and B. Gruenewald

Fritz-Haber-Institut der Max-Planck-Gesellschaft
Faradayweg 4-6, D-1000 Berlin 33,
West Germany

INTRODUCTION

Phospholipid-water assemblies are of great interest for purely
physico-chemical reasons as well as to contribute to our knowledge of
the correlation between structure and function in biological membranes.
More specialised applications of phospholipid aggregates are found in
food and foam technology and in selective drug transport.

Depending on the type of the polar headgroups (charged or
zwitterionic) and of the hydrocarbon chains (length and degree of
unsaturation) phospholipids show the tendency for self association
in water which is due to two different types of interactions, caused
on one hand by the hydrophilic headgroups and on the other hand by
the hydrophobic chains[1].

The phase-diagram in Fig. 1 contains the main types of molecular
assemblies which were found in aqueous solutions of di-palmitoyl-
phosphatidylcholine[2,3]. Simple macroscopic structures are obtained
only in very concentrated solutions (lamellar stacks of lipid bilayers)
or in very dilute solutions (single walled vesicles). In the intermediate range closed multilamellar aggregates like elongated tubes or
multishelled vesicles (liposomes) are formed; long-lived metastable
structures may be found, while the thermodynamic stable state is not
yet known. All these assemblies undergo structural phase transitions
initiated by temperature changes. The most important phase change is
the chain melting-transition (main transition, 40°C) which separates
the fluid (Lα) and the crystalline (Pβ,Lβ) phases. Here the hexagonal
order of the headgroups breaks down and the conformation of the hydrocarbon chains alters from an all trans order to a mixed cis-trans conformation. The pretransition which is only observed in large vesicles

185

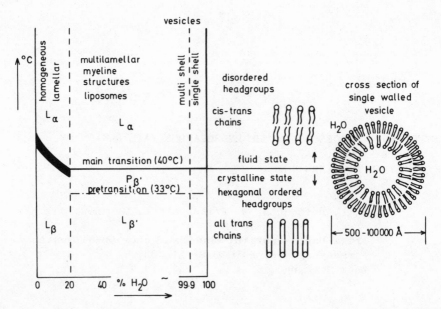

Fig. 1.   Phase diagram of dipalmitoyl-phosphatidylcholine (DPPC) as
suggested by x-ray[2] electron microscopy[3] and optical birefringence[18]. The broad black area is a region of coexistence. Small
single walled vesicles as indicated in the figure are normally
spheric. β indicates the crystalline phase while α stands for the
liquid phase.

and liposomes or myeline-structures can be explained by a spontaneous
curvature of the partly decoupled monolayers forming the bilayered
membranes[3].

     In addition to the above mentioned equilibrium and thermodynamic
properties of the phase transition, kinetic aspects have found relatively little consideration, which may partly be due to the apparent
complexity of the problem. Nonetheless, kinetic studies of vesicles
and liposomes may provide information for the dynamics of phospholipids in their membrane environment and their function both as a
fluidity switch and a passive transport barrier. Our dynamic investigations are therefore concentrated on single walled vesicles and
some preliminary kinetic studies of liposomes.

EXPERIMENTAL

Kinetic Methods

The complexity of the phase transition kinetics in vesicles is reflected by the spectrum of effects as observed with relaxation methods. Two groups of applied techniques are to be differentiated: ultrasonic and dielectric relaxation on one hand[4-8] as well as temperature-jump and pressure-jump relaxation[9-14] on the other. These dynamic investigations evidently have something to do with the properties of the phospholipid bilayer phase transition, but the interpretation on a molecular basis still lacks clarity. Here we concentrate on a special laser-temperature-jump and a pressure-jump method with observation of solution turbidity. Our results overcome three essential disadvantages of previous Joule-heating temperature jump experiments: 1. Dielectric breakdown of the lipid bilayer due to a transient electric field can be excluded[13,15-17]; no separate orientation effect on the lipid headgroups as again an electric field causes are occurring[7]. 2. The extremely fast time resolution of our laser-temperature jump of 1 nanosecond is independent of additives because the solvent water is heated through laser-photon absorption in vibrational rotational states. 3. Laser-temperature-jumps as well as pressure jumps provide isotropic conditions in the sense that temporarily different temperatures between inside and outside of vesicles are excluded[17].

Solution turbidity or scattered light intensity are frequently applied observation means for the phase transitions of one component phospholipid bilayers[19,20]. These methods yield relatively unspecific quantities in terms of structural information, but they offer the advantages of detection without labels which might change the molecular environment, and of easy applicability in kinetic experiments.

Laser Temperature Jump

A UV-flash induced dissociation reaction of the gas perfluoro-isopropyliodide ($i-C_3F_7J$) into $C_3F_7^*$ and J^* ($^2P_{\frac{1}{2}}$) is used for laser action (transition between $J^*(^2P_{\frac{1}{2}})$ and $J(^2P_{3/2})$)[21-23]. In detail this iodine laser was described previously[21-23]. From the emitted pulse train at 1.315 μm a single pulse is selected, amplified and passed through a quartz cuvette with the aqueous solution under investigation resulting in laser pulse half width of 0.6 - 3 nanoseconds depending on the mode of operation. The laser light energy is absorbed by rotational-vibrational states of the water molecules (the solvent) and converted into heat within a time equal to the duration of the laser pulse. This is due to the very short life-times of excited vibrational-rotational states in H_2O[24]. The conversion of energy results in a temperature jump of about 1K within an effective volume of ca. 40 μl in a quartz cuvette containing 500 μl sample solution. The cuvette was thermostated with an accuracy of $\pm$0.1 K.

Laser temperature-jumps were repeated about every three minutes within
which thermal equilibrium of the cuvette was reached.

Rectangular to the laser light beam the intensity attenuation of
365 nm light from a Xenon lamp (XBO 150 W) was detected. The lamp was
pulsed by discharging a capacitor bench of 60-80 V within 500 microseconds. This made possible the use of a very fast low noise photomultiplier[25] with a rise time of 0.6 nanoseconds which operates with
only five dynodes and therefore requires high lamp power. This lamp
pulse is induced simultaneously with the laser emission. Filters
before and a monochromator behind the sample made sure that only the
desired part of the detection light passed through the sample and was
detected by the photomultiplier tube (RCA 1P28). The signal was
passed through an active probe Tektronix P6201 (bandwidth 900 MHz) and
stored in the Tektronix transient digitizer 7912 AD equipped with the
plugins 7 A 13 and 7 B 92 (bandwidth $\geq$ 100 MHz, rise time 2.6 nanoseconds. The Tektronix 7912 AD was connected to a calculator Hewlett-
Packard 9845 S via the IEEE 488 bus. Several experiments were averaged at each temperature by means of the above mentioned calculator.
A schematic diagram of the experimental arrangement is given in Fig. 2
Fig. 3 shows the emission time of a typical laser-pulse used in these
kinetic measurements.

Pressure-Jump

The pressure-jump method with optical detection (turbidity in our
case) has been described previously[26]. In this method, static pressure is applied to the sample cell for time intervals long enough to
allow chemical equilibration at the elevated pressure level. The
pressure-jump back to ambient conditions is accomplished by bursting
a metal membrane which seals the autoclave. Bursting pressure was
chosen at 150 bar for the liposome solutions and 55 bar for the vesicle solutions. Reproducibility of the bursting pressure is $\pm 10\%$
which is a main source of error in the amplitude determination. Dead-
time of the instrument is given by the brass membrane bursting-time
of a maximum of 100 μs. For vesicle suspensions the temperature was
kept constant (± 0.1 K) during each experiment and lowered stepwise to
the next constant value.

Lipids

The lipid L-β, γ-dipalmitoyl-α-phosphatidylcholine (DPPC) was
purchased from Fluka, Switzerland; its chemical structure and conformation is given in Fig. 4. In thin-layer chromatography no impurity
was detected; therefore the substances were used without further
purification.

Preparation of Lipid Aggregates

For the preparation of multilamellar liposomes, 10 mg dimyris-

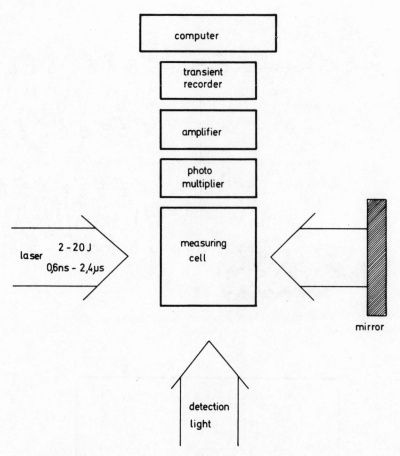

Fig. 2.   Schematic diagram of the laser-temperature jump arrangement
with time-resolution of 1ns.

toyl-phosphatidylcholine or dipalmitoyl-phosphatidylcholine were
sonicated for 1-2 min at low power in 10 ml bidistilled water at a
temperature above the corresponding phase transition temperature.
For each experiment a freshly prepared dispersion was used because
the suspensions tend to settle during longer times of standing.

Vesicles were prepared by injecting an ethanolic lipid solution
into the buffer at a temperature above the phase transition temperature (50°C) and subsequent dialysis against pure buffer for at least
8 h[15].   Buffer conditions were 0.01 M Tris-HCl (pH 7.5), 0.1 M NaCl
and 1 mM NaN_3.   The solution remains stable for several days if kept
at similar temperatures as during preparation.   This was tested by

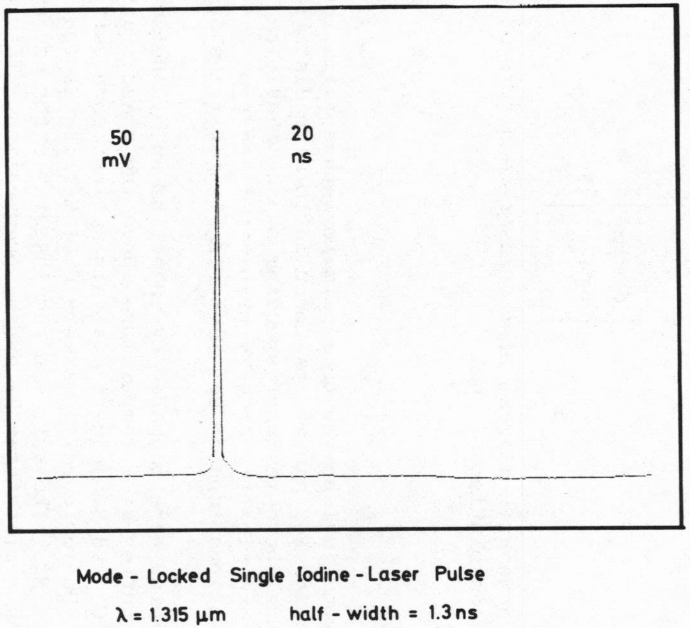

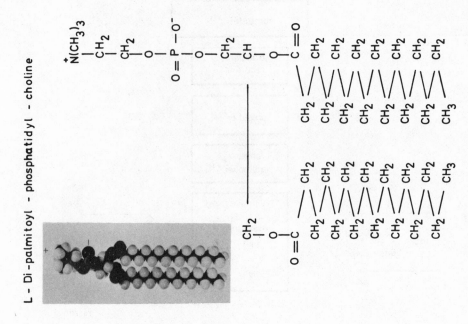

L - Di -palmitoyl - phosphatidyl - choline

Fig.4. Chemical bond structure and conformation model of DPPC.

Mode - Locked Single Iodine - Laser Pulse

λ = 1.315 μm   half - width = 1.3 ns

Fig. 3. Relaxation of the iodine-laser pulse
used for heating the samples; its half-width
is 1.3 ns.

measuring turbidity. In the case of vesicles the aggregate stability
towards pressure-jumps is a critical experimental point, because
breaking of the vesicles membrane into fragments might result in
reaggregation to large, potentially even multilayered structures. The
stability was checked by measuring the mean vesicle radii before and
after several pressure-jumps of 70 bar by means of the laser light
scattering autocorrelation technique. The mean vesicle radius proved
unaffected by the pressure perturbation. But from the dependence of
the correlation time on the sampling time it can be estimated that a
small portion of vesicles is broken up into fragments which reaggre-
gate to some unspecified species. Thus each pressure-jump is accompanied by a minute increase in solution turbidity. Undoubtedly this
affects the accuracy of the kinetic amplitudes for which reason we
chose to normalize these as described below. Since the steepness of
transition curves is a sensitive measure for the vesicle size[20] and
the integrated amplitudes agree with the thermodynamically obtained
transition curves quite well (see Results section) we trust that the
bulk of all vesicles retains its shape after the perturbation.

Thermotropic Transition Curve

Thermotropic transition curves were observed by measuring turbidity with a Perkin Elmer photometer or 90° light-scattering intensity
with a Farrand MKl fluorometer at 365 nm wavelength. The temperature
was scanned at $12 \text{ K} \cdot \text{h}^{-1}$ from high to low temperature in the case of
small single walled vesicles; the experimental results in Fig. 5 show
only the main phase transition at $40^{\circ}C$.

The pretransition, which can only be observed in solutions of
large multishelled vesicles (liposomes), showing a hysteresis effect
in the temperature region of this transition around $30^{\circ}C$ is demonstrated in Fig. 6; for details see reference (27).

Application of Relaxation Methods to Phase Transitions

In most experiments on structural transitions the degree of
transition θ, is an easily determinable quantity. In the case of a
simple isomeric transition $A \rightleftharpoons B$, θ is the following function of the
equilibrium constant s:

$$\theta = \frac{s}{1 + s} \qquad \qquad ...(1)$$

In complex systems like molecular aggregates composed of a large
number of elements with a nearest-neighbour interaction (cooperativity), intermediate states between 'all elements in A' and 'all elements in B' occur with a certain probability. In such systems, $\theta = f$
(s, ...). The equilibrium constant, s, is then interpreted as a
quantity describing the elementary process of propagation of struc-

DPPC vesicles (small)

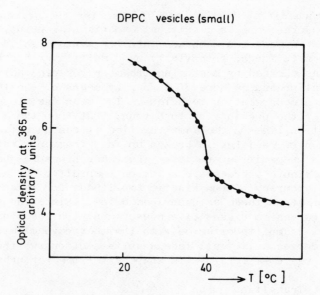

Fig. 5. Equilibrium phase transition curve of small single shelled vesicles of DPPC as measured by turbidity changes. Only one reversible transition is observed at 40°C.

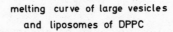

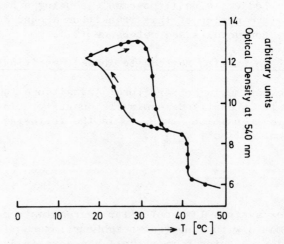

Fig. 6. Heating and cooling curve of liposomes of DPPC. A pronounced hysteresis is seen for the pretransition. Turbidity changes at 540 nm were measured because of the high optical density.

tural change, and the other parameters are, for instance, nucleation parameters and the number of elements. Since of all processes, propagation steps predominate with by far the highest probability of occurrence, the shift of Θ by means of temperature or pressure is, therefore, controlled practically by the equilibrium constant, s, alone. The dependence of Θ on s, however, may be complex. As an example, the application of the one-dimensional Ising model to helix-coil transitions can be mentioned[28,29].

For our kinetic experiments we need to know the amplitude $\delta\Theta$ as a function of s. At $P_o = 1$ atm, s is

$$s = \exp \left[- \frac{\Delta H^o}{RT} + \frac{\Delta S^o}{R} \right] = s_o(T) \qquad \ldots (2a)$$

and at $P \neq 1$ atm

$$s = s_o(T) \cdot \exp \left[- \frac{\Delta V^o}{RT} (P-P_o) \right] \qquad \ldots (2b)$$

For cooperative structural transitions, ΔH^o is equal to the calorimetrically determined molar transition enthalpy, ΔH_{cal}, and ΔV^o is equal to the molar transition volume as obtained from compressibility or density data. The amplitude $\delta\Theta$ can be taken from the following equations

$$\left(\frac{\partial \Theta}{\partial T} \right)_P = \Gamma \left(\frac{\partial \ln s}{\partial T} \right)_P = \Gamma \cdot \frac{\Delta H_{cal}}{RT^2} \qquad \ldots (3a)$$

or

$$\left(\frac{\partial \Theta}{\partial P} \right)_T = \Gamma \left(\frac{\partial \ln s}{\partial P} \right)_T = -\Gamma \cdot \frac{\Delta V^o}{RT} \qquad \ldots (3b)$$

For simplicity we set $\delta\Theta / \ln s = \Gamma$. In the case of a rapid pressure change, Eqn. 3b needs an amendment for the adiabatic temperature effect. The combination of Eqns. 3a and 3b yields

$$\left(\frac{\partial \Theta}{\partial P} \right)_T = - \left(\frac{\partial \Theta}{\partial T} \right)_P \cdot \frac{T \cdot \Delta V^o}{\Delta H_{cal}} \qquad \ldots (4)$$

This relation demonstrates the equivalence of temperature and pressure perturbation and represents a convenient tool for kinetic experiments on cooperative transitions. Without the knowledge of the

pressure induced transition curve (special equipment is necessary for
its determination), Eqn. 4 permits predictions about the amplitude
of pressure-jump experiments from the thermotropic transition alone.
For structural transitions Eqn. 4 also comprises an interesting parallel with the Clausius-Clapeyron relation for the coexistence curve
between two phases, 1 and 2, in a phase diagram:

$$\frac{T \cdot \Delta V^o}{\Delta H_{cal}} = (\frac{dT}{dP}) \qquad \qquad \dots (5)$$

Obviously the slopes of transition curves reach maxima at the
mid-point of transition. These maxima we define as $[\partial\Theta/\partial T]_{P-m}$ and
$[\partial/\partial P]_{T-m}$ and the corresponding amplitude factor as Γ_m. This mid-
point amplitude factor, Γ_m, can serve as a measure for the cooperativity of the investigated system. If we assume artificially a two-
state mechanism $A \rightleftharpoons B$ (which is never true for complex cooperative
transitions) the amplitude factor is given by $\Gamma = \Theta(1-\Theta)$ which is
0.25 for $\Theta = 0.5$. Thus, Eqns. 3a and 3b will read at the mid-point
of transition

$$(\frac{\partial\Theta}{\partial T})_{P,T_m} = \frac{\Delta H_{vH}}{4RT_m^2} \qquad \qquad \dots (6a)$$

and

$$(\frac{\partial\Theta}{\partial P})_{T,P_m} = -\frac{\Delta V_{vH}}{4RT} \qquad \qquad \dots (6b)$$

The van't Hoff quantities ΔH_{vH} and ΔV_{vH} are defined by these
equations. The real mechanism may imply $\Gamma \neq \Theta(1-\Theta)$. However, according to essentially all plausible models, Γ will assume a maximum Γ_m
at $\Theta = \frac{1}{2}$, i.e. T_m or P_m, and we find from the comparison between an
artificial two-state model (Eqns. 6a and 6b) and an unspecified real
mechanism (Eqns. 3a and 3b at mid-point conditions).

$$4\Gamma_m = \frac{\Delta H_{vH}}{\Delta H_{cal}} = \frac{\Delta V_{vH}}{\Delta V^o} \qquad \qquad \dots (7)$$

The ratio $\Delta H_{vH}/\Delta H_{cal}$ has frequently been used as a measure for
cooperativity[11,20]. Its close relation to the amplitude factor
Γ_m allows a decision about the extent of the observed cooperativity.
Evidently $4\Gamma_m = 1$ for a non-cooperative process.

Formation of Kinks in Vesicles of DPPC

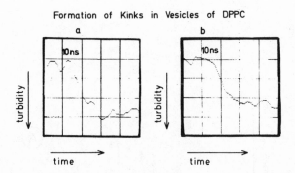

Fig. 7. (a) Turbidity (increase) relaxation of DPPC-vesicles at 43°C, observed in a single temperature-jump experiment. The grid unit corresponds to 10 nanoseconds. (b) Same specifications as for (a), but four experiments were superimposed and averaged. Relaxation time equal to 5 nanoseconds.

RESULTS

We report relaxation results on single walled vesicles of DPPC in the nanosecond time range initiated by temperature jumps and measurements in the microsecond-millisecond time region investigated with pressure jumps. Relaxation curves were obtained for the temperature range of 30°C - 46°C including the DPPC main phase-transition temperature T_m = 40°C. The very fast relaxation proceeds with an increase of solution turbidity within the investigated time interval. The relaxation time of this effect was determined as τ_{VF} = 4±0.5 nanoseconds without a significant dependence on temperature, especially without a pronounced maximum at the transition midpoint T_m. In Fig. 7a single relaxation curve and an average over four signals is given. A least square fit of the signal between 3 ns and 20 ns results in a relaxation time of 5±0.5 ns. If we take into account the influence of the electronic detection circuit we calculate the real relaxation time as 4±0.5 nanoseconds. At the phase transition temperature, T_m, we find a small increase in the amplitude of 10-20%, but this result is not pronounced enough to rely upon it. Further experiments are necessary to decide how much the amplitude is exactly changing at T_m.

Our kinetic results on DPPC vesicles measured with the pressure jump technique are shown in Fig. 8a,b together with a normalized static transition curve for the main transition at T_m in Fig. 8c; for details see reference[30]. For all solutions we observed two distinct relaxation effects which showed a decrease in turbidity: a fast relaxation (τ_F) around 300 microseconds, and a slow one (τ_s)

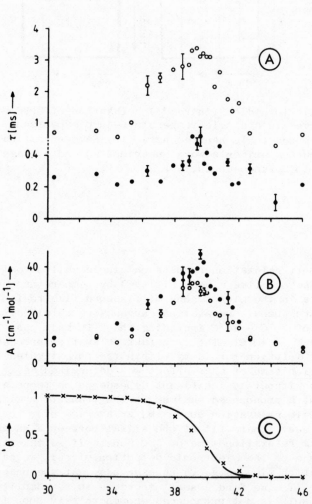

Fig. 8. Pressure-jump experiments on dipalmitoyl-phosphatidylcholine
(DPPC) vesicles of 25 nm radius. Lipid concentrations was 2 mM in
0.1 M NaCl/0.01 M Tris.HCl (pH 7.5)/1 mM NaN$_3$. a) Relaxation times
as a function of temperature, o, slow effect; •, fast effect.
b) Relaxation amplitudes from turbidity change at 365 nm after
pressure-jumps of 55 bar. The symbols correspond to those of (a).
c) Normalized transition curve (solid line) as obtained from light
scattering at 365 nm. Crosses represent numerical integration of
the amplitudes of (b) according to Eqn. 7.

around 2 milliseconds. Both of these phenomena are clearly associated
with the phase transition as the peaked τ versus T dependence demonstrates. To exclude the possibility of aggregation from these two
processes, we tested the concentration dependence of τ by diluting the
same preparation and thereby leaving the aggregates' dimensions
unchanged. Neither of the two relaxations exhibited different time
constants. Further evidence for the close relation between the observed processes, reflected in τ_F and τ_S, and the main phase transition
can be drawn from the good agreement between the thermotropic transition curve in Fig. 8c and the integrated sums of the pressure jump
amplitudes of τ_F and τ_S plotted as crosses in Fig. 8c. Details of
the integration are given in reference[30]. However, for reasons
which are explained in the experimental section, the amplitude determination remains relatively uncertain.

The characteristics of the very fast nanosecond relaxation times
(τ_{VF}) and amplitudes are quite contrary to the ones of the fast microsecond (τ_F) and the slower millisecond (τ_S) effects. In the former
turbidity increases with increasing temperature and exhibits the characteristics of noncooperativity (no pronounced maxima of τ_{VF} and
amplitude around T_m); in the latter turbidity decreases with increasing pressure and cooperativity is clearly demonstrated around T_m.
These points will be essential for the design of our model which is
presented in the following discussion.

DISCUSSION

The present results in combination with those from ultrasonic
absorption on lipid bilayers as obtained by a number of other authors
[5 - 8,31] allow the partial design of a model for the phase transition of lipid membranes. In the following this will be introduced and
discussed in the light of the available experimental data.

Our model is schematically drawn in Fig. 9. It is assumed that
the phase transition proceeds with a sequence of steps. Upon raising
the temperature (or lowering the pressure) at first a structural
change is induced in the chains of a number of lipid molecules. This
process is accomplished within at most 10 nanoseconds and represents
the formation of rotational isomers (e.g. kinks, as introduced by
Träuble and Haynes[32] and Seelig and Seelig[33]). It has maximal
probability of occurrence in the midpoint of transition. The time of
10 nanoseconds does not suffice, however, to install the new equilibrium state of the membrane. The completion of the new state requires
at least an expansion of the membrane to a larger surface area per
molecule, a smaller bilayer thickness and an increase of the internal
vesicular volume surrounded by the membrane[34-36]. The steps between
the formation of rotational isomers and the completion of the new
equilibrium include cooperative processes on a much longer time scale
than the initial "kink-step"[13,30,37]. The nature of the two slower
steps, however, seems to be rather complicated and can be attributed

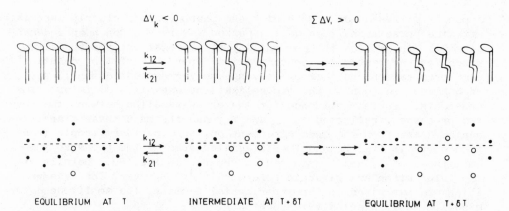

Fig. 9.   Schematic arrangements of lipid molecules in the hexagonal lattice of a bilayer: ● molecules in the solid state, o molecules in the fluid state. From left to right the scheme depicts the stepwise assumption of a new equilibrium state induced by a rise of temperature The broken line represents a vertical cut through the bilayer. The molecules bordering this cut are shown with the appropriate structure above the lattice.

to changes in the whole membrane structure. The observed very fast effects are concentration independent. That they are intramolecular processes rather than rearrangements within the aggregate structure is plausible for two reasons. First we did not detect any dependence of relaxation times on the type of the lipid aggregate (vesicle or liposome) contrary to the μs- and ms-effects[30]. And second even a dramatic change of lipid head group structure like the introduction of a charge, as done by Hammes and Roberts[31] by measuring ultrasonic absorption on phosphatidyl-serine, does not change the time range of relaxation.

We find our experiment and interpretation reconfirmed by the fact that the correlation time for the rotational motion of lipid chain segments was measured to be between 10 and 100 picoseconds by deuterium NMR[38]. It should be noted, however, that turbidity detects an overall process and is not specific. Changes in the location of the head groups which occur on the same time scale as our turbidity changes may also contribute to our sigaal[39-43], but is not inferred in our model.

The formation of a kink within a time interval in which the environment of the converting molecule cannot accommodate the need for the required space, implies a local shrinkage of bilayer thickness and

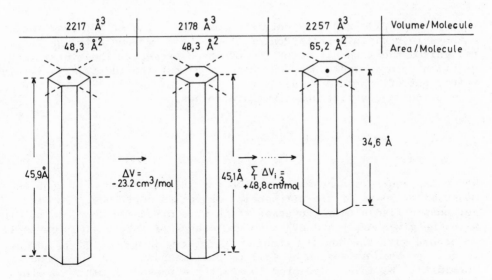

| 2217 $\overset{\circ}{A}^3$ | 2178 $\overset{\circ}{A}^3$ | 2257 $\overset{\circ}{A}^3$ | Volume/Molecule |
| 48,3 $\overset{\circ}{A}^2$ | 48,3 $\overset{\circ}{A}^2$ | 65,2 $\overset{\circ}{A}^2$ | Area/Molecule |

45,9Å $\Delta V = -23.2 \, cm^3/mol$ 45,1Å $\sum_i \Delta V_i = +48,8 \, cm^3/mol$ 34,6 Å

EQUILIBRIUM AT T   INTERMEDIATE AT T+δT   EQUILIBRIUM AT T+δT

Fig. 10. Schemes of the molecular volume of lipids in the hexagonal
lattice of a bilayer: no kink at T, kink at T + δT without expansion
of the environment, kink at the new equilibrium state. The dot in
the hexagonal place represents the position of the vertical glycerol
backbone. See the text for the indicated quantities.

simultaneous increase of density. This agrees with the observation
of turbidity increase after the fast temperature-jump since turbidity
is proportional to the fourth power (for point scatterers) of the
refractive index, n, which in turn increases monotonously with density
[19]. Another source of increasing turbidity could be an increase of
molecular anisotropy[19]. This possibility is disregarded, however,
because to our knowledge there is no evidence for rise of order with
rising temperature.

The local shrinkage is visualized crudely in Fig. 10. If we
assume a hexagonal prism for the molecular volume with a cross section
of 48.3 Å(39) and further a kink to cause a shortening of the lipid
chain within the same cross section by about 0.8 Å, we obtain a reac-
tion volume for the kink formation of 38.6 $\overset{\circ}{A}^3$ per molecule or $\Delta V_k =$
-23.2 cm^3/mol. From the amplitude of ultrasonic absorption of
DPPC-vesicles Gamble and Schimmel (6) calculated $\Delta V = 24.6 \pm 3.0 \, cm^3/$
mol in good accord with our picture.

The circumstance, however, that the ultrasonic absorption amplitude yields $(\Delta V)^2$ and thus only the absolute value of ΔV, lead those authors to a misinterpretation of the reaction volume although they recognized the true nature of the observed process. The overall reaction volume namely happens to be of almost the identical absolute value, but of opposite sign: $\Delta V_{tot} = +24.2$ cm^3/mol [44,45]. In the view of our sequential model we have to assume

$$\Delta V_{tot} = \Delta V_k + \Sigma \Delta V_i \qquad \qquad \ldots (8)$$

where ΔV_k equals the reaction volume for the formation of a kink as measured by means of the ultrasonic absorption amplitude. For the yet unspecified slower processes which were discussed above we obtain with the given ΔV_{tot} and ΔV_k a volume change of $\Sigma \Delta V_i = +48.8$ cm^3/mol. In accord with the density changes during the progress of the phase transition this expansion by 48.8 cm^3/mol means a strong decrease of turbidity. We indeed detected this after a pressure-jump from elevated pressure to 1 atm (which corresponds to an upwards temperature-jump) [30].

From our laser temperature-jump experiments we find no dependence of the relaxation time τ_{VF} on the temperature. An Arrhenius-dependence with a very small activation energy ought to be hidden in the experimental uncertainty. Since we do not observe a clear maximum of τ_{VF} in the midpoint of transition we assume that the observed process is an isomerization independent of molecular interactions within the membrane lattice. We can thus write for the relaxation rate

$$\frac{1}{\tau_{VF}} = k_{12} + k_{21} \qquad \qquad \ldots (9)$$

For the midpoint of transition the equilibrium constant

$$K = \frac{k_{12}}{k_{21}} \qquad \qquad \ldots (10)$$

must be unity and therefore $k_{12} = k_{21}$. Hence the respective rate is $1/\tau_m = 2 k_{12}$. With a relaxation time of 4 ns we obtain $k_{12}^{40o} = k_{21}^{40o} = 1.25 \times 10^8$ s^{-1}. This agrees satisfactorily with the data of Gamble and Schimmel [6] from whom $k_{12}^{40o} = k_{21}^{40o} = 5.10^7$ s^{-1} is calculated.

A comparison between the described ns-processes occurring in the hydrophobic tail region of the lipid bilayer and kinetic processes in small or large chain molecules (alcanes, vinylic polymers) reveals

that the rate of rotation about C-C-bonds does not depend drastically
on the environment as long as hydrocarbon chains are considered in a
hydrophobic environment. For polystyrene in various organic solvents
relaxation times between 10 and 50 nanoseconds were obtained from
ultrasonic absorption[46,47]. Even a variation of solvent viscosity
by a factor of 50 changed the relaxation time only by a factor of 3[48].
Ultrasonic relaxation in higher liquid n-alkanes n = 9...14 yielded
relaxation times of 30-70 nanoseconds and showed that shorter chains
rotate slightly faster than longer ones[49].

        Also we want to emphasize some parallels between the dynamic
behaviours of liquid crystals and lipid bilayers. Jähnig[50] showed
that for MBBA in the neighbourhood of the nematic-isotropic phase
transition the anisotropic attenuation of ultrasound is caused by two
superposing effects: intramolecular trans-gauche rotations and the
relaxation of the nematic order parameter. If the ultrasound frequency
is chosen small enough these two contributions to the anisotropic
sound attenuation are proportional to the respective relaxation times.
The one for the C-C-bond rotations, τ_i, exhibits an Arrhenius temperature dependence with an activation energy of 17.6 kJ/mol and the relaxation of the order parameter has a time constant τ_c with a critical
increase in the neighbourhood of the phase transition. The rotational
relaxation time τ_i was found to be 20 nanoseconds at 298 K. The interpretation of the effects with a "critical" relaxation behaviour appears
to be more complex for vesicles and liposomes than for liquid crystals
because two effects instead of only one are observed[13,30]. However,
the similarity between the observations on the ns-effects supports the
concept of a close relationship for the fast C-C-bond rotations in
both systems. At last a word is to be said about whether kinks in a
lipid chain actually migrate with this chain. Diffusion coefficients
D were obtained mainly by NMR and ESR and yielded values around D =
10^{-8} cm^2/s in the fluid state of the membrane[51]. The expression

$$D = \frac{<\lambda^2>}{4}$$

...(11)

($<\lambda^2>$ = mean of the square of jump distance or distance between two
bilayer lattice points, τ = mean time lag between two jumps of a molecule from one lattice point to another) which is derived for a two
dimensional random walk, may serve for a crude comparison of time constants. The time lag obtained from the mentioned diffusion coefficients is then 190 nanoseconds if λ is assumed to be 8.7 Å. This time
constant can be considered a lower limit since it was calculated for
the fluid state. The result of this present work is that kink formation requires less than 10 nanoseconds time. This means that lipid
molecules assume and lose kinks while they reside at any picked lattice point. Different energetic states like chains with kinks and
chains without kinks are therefore forwarded through the lattice
preferentially by energetic transitions which are handed on from one

molecule to another. The hypothesis of a migration of individual
molecules carrying a fixed energetic state can now be excluded. The
translation of energetic states ought to be considered as a cooperative
process and the growth and shrinkage of clusters of states ought to
be seen in this light.

ACKNOWLEDGEMENT

We wish to thank the Deutsche Forschungsgemeinschaft, Bonn, for
financial support.

REFERENCES

1.   C. Tanford, They Hydrophobic Effect, Wiley, New York 1973.
2.   D. Chapman, R. M. Williams and B. D. Ladbrooke, Chem. Phys.
     Lipids 1, 445 (1967).
3.   C. Gebhardt, H. Gruler, and E. Sackmann, Z. Naturforschung
     32c, 581 (1977).
4.   U. Kaatze, R. Henze, A. Seegers and R. Pottel, Ber. Bunsenges.
     Physik. Chem. 79, 42. (1975).
5.   F. Eggers, and Th. Funck, Naturwissenschaften 63, 280, (1976).
6.   R. C. Gamble and P. R. Schimmel, Proc. Natl. Acad. Sci. U.S.A.
     75, 3011 (1978).
7.   J. C. W. Shepherd and G. Büldt, Biochim. Biophys. Acta 514, 83,
     (1978).
8.   J. E. Harkness and R. D. White Biochim. Biophys. Acta 552, 450,
     (1979).
9.   G. G. Hammes, and D. E. Tallman, J. Am. Chem. Soc. 92, 6042,
     (1970).
10. J. D. Owen, P. Hemmes, and E. M. Eyring Biochim. Biophys. Acta
     219, 276, (1970).
11. H. Traüble, Naturwissenschaften 58, 277, (1971).
12. T. Y. Tsong, Proc. Natl. Acad. Sci. U.S.A. 71, 2684 (1974).
13. T. Y. Tsong and M. I. Kanehisa, Biochemistry 16, 2674 (1977).
14. R. M. Clegg, E. L. Elson and B. W. Maxfield, Biopolymers 14,
     883 (1975).
15. T. Y. Tsong, T. T. Tsong, E. Kingsley and R. Siliciano, Biophys.
     J. 14, 881 (1974).
16. U. Zimmermann, G. Pilwat and F. Riemann, Biophys. J. 14, 881,
     (1974).
17. J. D. Owen, B. C. Bennion, L. P. Holmes, E. M. Eyring,
     M. W. Berg, and J. L. Lords, Biochim. Biophys. Acta 203, 77
     (1970).
18. L. Powers and P. S. Pershan, Biophys. J. 20, 137 (1977).
19. P. N. Yi, and R. C. MacDonald, Chem. Phys. Lipids 11, 114, (1975).
20. B. Gruenewald, S. Stankowski, and A. Blume, FEBS Letters 102, 227,
     (1979).
21. J. F. Holzwarth, A. Schmidt, H. Wolff and R. Volk, J. Phys. Chem.
     81, 2300 (1977).

22. J. F. Holzwarth, in: Techniques and Applications of Fast Reactions in Solution (W. J. Gettins, and E. Wyn-Jones, eds.), Reidel, Dordrecht, 61-70 (1979).

23. W. Frisch, A. Schmidt, J. F. Holzwarth and R. Volk, in: Techniques and Applications of Fast Reactions in Solution (W. J. Gettins and E. Wyn-Jones, E., eds.), Reidel, Dordrecht, 61-70 (1979).

24. D. M. Gooddall and R. C. Greenhow, Chem. Phys. Letters 9, 583, (1971).

25. G. Beck Rev. Sci. Instrum. 47, 537 (1976).

26. B. Gruenewald, and W. Knoche, in: Techniques and Applications of Fast Reactions in Solution (W. J. Gettins, and E. Wyn-Jones, eds.) Reidel, Dordrecht (1979).

27. T. Y. Tsong and M. I. Kanehisa, Biochemistry 16, 2674 (1977).

28. B. H. Zimm and J. K. Bragg J. Chem. Phys. 31, 526 (1959).

29. G. Schwarz J. Mol. Biol. 11, 64 (1965).

30. B. Gruenewald, A. Blume and F. Watanabe, Biochim, Biophys. Acta 597, 41 (1980).

31. G. G. Hammes and P. B. Roberts Biochim. Biophys. Acta 203, 220, (1970).

32. H. Träuble and D. H. Haynes Chem. Phys. Lipids 7, 324 (1971).

33. A. Seelig and J. Seelig Biochemistry 13, 4839 (1974).

34. A. Tardieu, V. Luzzatti and F. C. Reman J. Mol. Biol. 75, 711, (1973).

35. M. J. Janiak, D. M. Small and G. G. Shipley, Biochemistry 15, 4575 (1976).

36. A. Watts, D. Marsh and P. F. Knowles, Biochemistry 17, 1792 (1978).

37. J. Teissie, Biochim. Biophys. Acta 555, 553 (1979).

38. M. F. Brown, J. Seelig and U. Häberlen, J. Chem. Phys. 70, 5045, (1979).

39. J. C. W. Shepherd and G. Büldt, Biochim. Biophys. Acta 514, 83 (1979).

40. J. C. W. Shepherd and G. Büldt, Biochim. Biophys. Acta 558, 41 (1979).

41. U. Kaatze, R. Henze, A. Seegers and R. Pottel Ber. Bunsenges, 79, 42 (1975).

42. U. Kaatze, R. Henze and R. Pottel, Chem Phys. Lipids 25, 149 (1979).

43. U. Kaatze, R. Henze and H. Eibl, Biophys. Chem. 10, 351 (1979).

44. K. R. Srinivasan, R. L. Kay and J. F. Nagle, Biochemistry 13, 3494 (1974).

45. N. I. Liu and R. L. Kay Biochemistry 16, 3484 (1977).

46. H. J. Bauer, H. Hässler and M. Immendörfer Disc. Faraday Soc. 49, 238 (1970).

47. K. Ono, H. Shintani, O. Yano and Y. Wada, Polymer J. 5, 164 (1973).

48. H. Ott, R. Cerf., B. Michels, and P. Lemarechal, Chem. Phys. Letters 24, 323 (1974).

49. M. A. Cochran, P. B. Jones, A. M. North and R. A. Pethrick, J. Chem. Soc., Faraday Transact. II 1719-1728 (1972).

50. J. Jähnig, Chem. Phys. Letters 23, 262, (1973).
51. A. G. Lee, Progr. Biophys. Molec. Biol. 29, 3 (1975).

DISCUSSION

Dr. A. Höhener: Do you have any idea where the kinks occur along the
chains?

Dr. J. F. Holzwarth: From our experiment we cannot decide in which
part of the hydrocarbon chain the observed rotational isomers (kinks)
are occurring, because the parameter turbidity which we used to follow
the relaxation curve is not specific enough. NMR measurements are
suitable to decide whether those kinks are formed near the headgroups
or if they mainly appear in the following part of the hydrocarbon
chains.

The present knowledge concerning this question is that there
exists a distribution of kinks over the whole hydrocarbon chains. The
measurements of J. Seelig on DPPC (Quarterly Review of Biophysics
(1977) 10,3 pp. 395-397) show a plateau of the order parameter in the
region of the first nine carbon atoms (near the headgroups) and a
decrease of the order (increase of the probability of kink formation)
with increasing slope towards the end of the hydrocarbon chains.

Dr. I. D. Robb: Why does kink formation lead to an increase in turbidity if the vesicle does not expand?

Dr. J. F. Holzwarth: Our measuring parameter turbidity is a complex
quantity; it is mainly determined by the local density and the order
inside the membrane, not by its size, if we look at aggregates like
vesicles with a phospholipid bilayer around a water pool of some
hundred $\overset{o}{A}$ in diameter. The formation of a kink within a time interval of some nanoseconds in which the environment of the chain now
containing a kink cannot accommodate the need for the required space,
implies a local shrinkage of bilayer thickness and simultaneous
increase of density. Turbidity is proportional to the fourth power
of the refractive index, n, which in turn increases monotonously with
density. The possibility of an increase of turbidity as well is
disregarded, because to our knowledge there is no evidence for rise
of order with rising temperature in bilayers of DPPC. For details of
scattering theory see Yi, P. N. and MacDonald, R. C. (1975) Chem.
Phys. Lipids 11, pp. 114-134.

Dr. B. H. Robinson: Can this technique be applied to other systems,
like microemulsions?

Dr. J. F. Holzwarth: In our temperature-jump technique we use an
iodine-laser as heating source. This laser emits photons at a wavelength of 1.315 μm. These photons are absorbed by combined overtone

vibrational-rotational states of OH-bonds, in our case by water. The heating time is therefore similar to the laser-emission time, approximately 1 nanosecond. In microemulsions water droplets are surrounded by amphiphilic molecules forming aggregates which are solved in an oil-like environment. This microstructure is the reason why I think that our technique is especially suitable for temperature-jump experiments which are performed to observe relaxation signals due to changes of the equilibrium inside the water droplets. If we consider possible effects on a time scale, the following can be expected: in the nanosecond region we expect relaxation signals due to changes inside the water pools. In the microsecond region temperature equilibration with the surrounding solution has to be considered. How fast the new temperature equilibrium of the whole solution is reached depends on the size, the number per cubic centimeter and the distance of the water pools. But some important advantages of our technique in comparison with the conventional Joule-heating arrangements should be mentioned: (1) Our heating time is independent of additives, especially of the ionic content of a solution; (2) in Joule-heating experiments the necessary high electric field which precedes the temperature-jump and relaxes with the increase of temperature will certainly affect the shape and structure of the water pools in the microemulsion; this field effect causes additional relaxations as well as serious optical artifacts which can be completely avoided with our technique. The only prerequisite for our temperature-jump experiment is the existence of OH-bonds, preferably in the major part of the solution which is normally the solvent.

Prof. Dr. H. F. Eicke: Do the vesicles respond reversibly to the applied temperature-jump experiments?

Dr. J. F. Holzwarth: We have tested the reversibility of our temperature-jump experiments in two ways: (1) the amplitudes of different single measurements following each other every three minutes initiated at the same temperature, caused by equivalent temperature increases, were equal within the accuracy of the experiment ($\pm 10\%$); (2) solution turbidity which can be used as a measure for the size and type of the vesicles (single-shelled or multi-shelled aggregates) was tested before and after each series of experiment, no changes could be detected.

We know that in Joule-heating temperature-jump experiments such a behaviour is difficult to be achieved. This is mainly due to possible membrane fracture caused by the high electric field (see also answer to Dr. Robinson) applied in this technique. In those experiments the membrane fracture might be followed by the formation of larger vesicles or liposomes, which changes turbidity. Small temperature-jumps and sufficient time for self-healing might possibly avoid the formation of larger aggregates, but special care has to be taken.

PROPERTIES OF HIGH EMULSIFIER CONTENT O/W MICROEMULSIONS

R. A. Mackay

Department of Chemistry
Drexel University
Philadelphia, PA 19104
U.S.A.

INTRODUCTION

We have been interested for some time in the use of microemulsions as solvents and media for the investigation of chemical reactions and interactions between oil and water soluble species[1]. Recently, other investigators have reported reaction studies in both O/W[2] and W/O[3] microemulsions. As a complimentary and necessary component of this work, some knowledge of the physical chemical properties of the systems employed must be obtained. Such properties are obtained by means of thermodynamic (phase maps, effective pH, component activity), transport (conductance, diffusion) and structural (light scattering, ultracentrifugation, dielectric, NMR) measurements. This list is not meant to be inclusive, and a number of other techniques have been brought to bear on the problem, such as microscopy[4], neutron scattering[5], etc.

In earlier studies, we examined the conductance of salt (NaCl) and the diffusion of Cd(II) in oil in water (O/W) microemulsions stabilized by nonionic surfactants[6]. In this paper we report additional data on nonionic systems, and the extension of these transport measurements to ionic O/W microemulsions.

EXPERIMENTAL

The conductivity measurements were performed using a dip cell containing platinized platinum electrodes (cell constant ~ 1) in conjunction with a Serfass conductance bridge operating at 1kHz. A Beckman Electroscan 30 and a three compartment cell was used for the dc polarographic measurements. The auxillary and reference electrodes

were platinum and saturated calomel (SCE), respectively. The solutions were deoxygenated by purging with nitrogen for at least 15 minutes. A bubbler containing microemulsion was used to prevent composition changes. A dropping mercury electrode and a rotating platinum
electrode were employed for the Cd(II) and $Fe(CN)_6^{3-/4-}$ ions, respectively. Viscosity measurements were performed with a thermostated
Ostwald viscometer tube calibrated with several pure fluids covering
the viscosity range of interest (1-100cp). Phase maps of the Tween
$40^{[7]}$, Tween $60^{[6]}$, and SCS$^{[8]}$ microemulsions have been published. A
newer phase map of the SCS system, showing a typical dilution line,
is presented in Fig. 1.

RESULTS AND DISCUSSION

Nonionic Microemulsions

       Previously, we showed[6] that the conductivity of nonionic micro-
emulsions containing added salt could be represented by equation (i),

$$\Lambda = \Lambda_o (1 - a\phi_{comp})^n \qquad\qquad (i)$$

where Λ and Λ_o are the equivalent conductivities in microemulsion
and water, respectively. The phase volume fraction calculated by
assuming the disperse phase consists of the surfactant, cosurfactant
(alcohol) and oil is given by $\phi_{comp} = 1 - \omega g$, where ω is the weight
fraction water and g is the specific gravity of the microemulsion.
The value of the parameter a was about 1.2 for the polyoxyethylene
surfactants examined and was interpreted as the contribution of water
associated with the drop to the phase volume (ϕ). The a value of 1.2
corresponded to 1-2 water molecules per ethylene oxide group. The
exponent n was 1.5 at low oil content, and decreased with increasing
oil content toward the value of 0.5 expected for a coarse emulsion.
The value of n was shown to correlate linearly with droplet diameter[9]
Although the microemulsion is concentrated in terms of phase volume
and total salt content, the equivalent conductance is essentially
independent of salt concentration. We therefore applied Walden's
Rule ($\Lambda\eta$ = constant), where η is the viscosity, to the continuous
phase of the microemulsion. This results in an expression for an
effective relative viscosity ($\eta_{r,eff}$) given by equation (ii).

$$\eta_{r,eff} = (1 - \phi)^{-(n+1)} \qquad\qquad (ii)$$

       Since the diffusion coefficient (D) of a species in the aqueous
phase should be inversely proportional to η, eq. (ii) predicts that
D should be given by equation (iii),

$$D = D_o (1 - \phi)^{n+1} \qquad\qquad (iii)$$

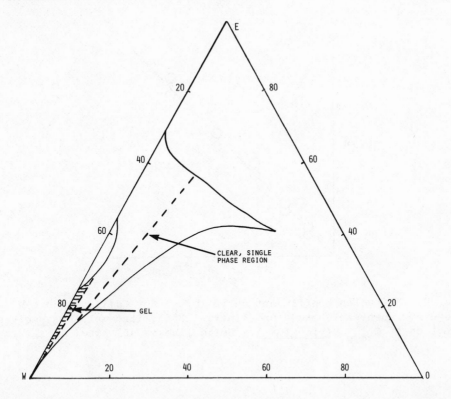

Fig. 1. Pseudo-three component phase map of the system emulsifier E (40% SCS, 60% 1-pentanol), water (W), and heavy mineral oil (O), by weight.

where D_0 is the diffusion coefficient in the continuous phase (water). This relationship was confirmed by polarographic measurement of the diffusion coefficient of Cd(II) ion in low oil content (initial 7% W/W) Tween 40 (10) and Tween 60 (6) microemulsions. The best fit was obtained for $n = 1.5$ and a value of D_0 corresponding to that of Cd(II) in water. The only difference between the diffusion and conductance results is that the value of ϕ_{comp} was used for the former. In order to explore the generality of this relationship, we performed additional measurements using other electroactive ions and Cd(II) at higher oil content. These measurements are discussed below.

Diffusion Coefficients of Aqueous ions in Nonionic Microemulsions

As discussed above, the exponent n obtained from conductivity measurements decreases with increasing oil content. Along the water dilution line in the Tween 60/1-pentanol/hexadecane system defined

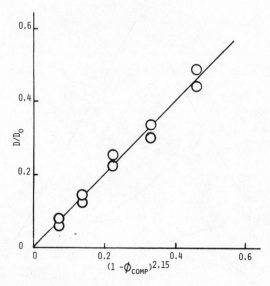

Fig. 2. Diffusion coefficient ratio (D/D_o) for Cd(II) in an O/W Tween 60/1-pentanol/hexadecane (initial 25%) microemulsion <u>vs</u> given function of ϕ_{comp}. (<u>vide text</u>). Solid line is 45° line.

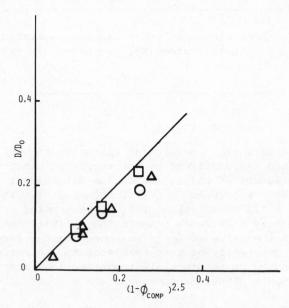

Fig. 3. Diffusion coefficient ratio (D/D_o) for Cd(II) (triangles), Fe(CN)$_6^{3-}$ (squares) and Fe(CN)$_6^{4-}$ (circles) in the Tween 40/1-pentanol/hexadecane (initial 7%) microemulsion <u>vs</u> given function of phase volume (<u>vide text</u>). Solid line is 45° line.

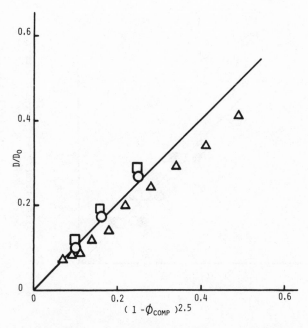

Fig. 4. Diffusion coefficient ratio (D/D_o) for Cd(II) (triangles), $Fe(CN)_6^{3-}$ (squares) and $Fe(CN)_6^{4-}$ (circles) in the Tween 60/1-pentanol/hexadecane (initial 7%) microemulsion vs given function of phase volume (vide text). Solid line is $45°$ line.

by the weight fraction oil (ω_o) to phase volume ratio $\omega_o/\phi=0.25$ (initial oil content of 25% W/W), a value of $n = 1.15$ is obtained from conductivity[6]. The diffusion coefficient ratio D/D_o for Cd(II) along the same dilution line vs $(1-\phi_{comp})^{(2.15)}$ is shown in Fig. 2. The data represent two independent sets of measurements. As can be seen from the figure, the agreement is excellent.

We have also measured values of D for both ferri- and ferrocyanide ions in both the Tween 40 and Tween 60 microemulsions at low (7% initial) oil content. The results are shown in Fig. 3 and Fig. 4, respectively. The previously reported values for Cd(II) are included for comparison. The agreement is again quite good and gives credence to the generality of equation (iii) and the transferability of the exponent n between diffusion and conductivity data. It should also be noted that, along with other lines of evidence, the D_o value indicates that the composition of the continuous (aqueous) phase of these O/W microemulsions is essentially that of plain water. This is in contrast to the situation in W/O microemulsions where the continuous (oil) phase contains significant amounts of alcohol cosurfactant.

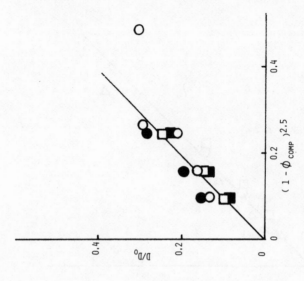

Fig. 6. Diffusion coefficient ratio (D/D_o) vs given function of phase volume for Tl(I) (open circles), Cd(II) (closed circles), Fe(CN)$_6^{3-}$ (open squares) and Fe(CN)$_6^{4-}$ (closed squares) in a 60% water/SCS/pentanol/mineral oil microemulsion (vide text). The solid line is the 45° line.

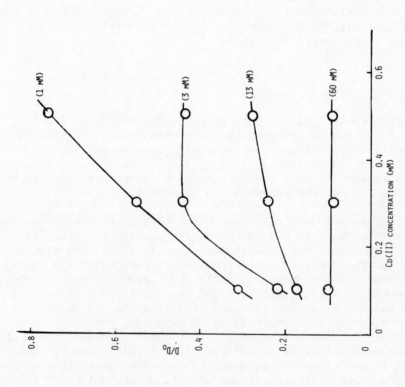

Fig. 5. Diffusion coefficient ratio (D/D_o) of Cd(II) vs Cd(II) concentration in aqueous solutions containing the specified concentration of SDS. The CMC of SDS is about 8mM.

Diffusion Coefficients of Ions in Ionic Microemulsions

In microemulsion systems stabilized by ionic surfactants, an aqueous ion of opposite charge may be fully or partially bound to the microdroplet surface. For example, Novodoff, Rosano, and Hoyer[11] employed Cd(II) ion as a tracer to measure the diffusion coefficient of aqueous sodium dodecyl sufate (SDS) micelles. Measurements such as these must be interpreted with care since Cd(II) cannot only bind to but also influence aqueous anionic micelles as shown in Fig. 5. However, these and other[11] results leave little doubt that the divalent cation is bound to the micelle. We have examined Cd(II) as well as Tl(I), $Fe(CN)_6^{3-}$ and $Fe/CN)_6^{4-}$ in an O/W sodium cetyl sulfate (SCS)/1-pentanol/mineral oil microemulsion, and the results are given in Fig. 6. Except for the Cd(II) point at low ϕ, which is near the phase boundary, all of the anion and cation diffusion coefficients behave as in a nonionic system. This might be expected for the anions but not for the cations, especially divalent Cd(II), which would be expected to be bound. In the 60% water SCS microemulsion, the concentration of droplets is on the order of 1mM(8), and both the half-wave potential and diffusion coefficient for Cd(II) is constant within experimental error ($\pm 10\%$) over a cadmium concentration range of 0.1 - 10 mM. We therefore conclude that the transport of all of the above ions in the ionic microemulsion is governed by movement through the aqueous phase. The cations are either not bound, perhaps due to the lower surface potential of microdrops compared with micelles, or are only weakly bound.

By way of contrast, we have also examined the water insoluble 1-dodecyl-4-cyanopyridinium ion in the SCS microemulsion. Over water contents ranging from 35 - 65%, the value of D was constant at a value of $4.4\pm0.4 \times 10^{-7}$ cm^2s^{-1}. From the Stokes-Einstein equation $D = kT/6\pi\eta r$, a hydrodynamic radius of 45Å is calculated using the viscosity of water. This may be compared with a value of 50Å obtained from low angle x-ray(8). Thus, oil soluble species appear to diffuse with the drop. Some very preliminary measurements with a cationic microemulsion, as well as with other probes, are in accord with this conclusion. If confirmed by future experiments, this provides a convenient method for obtaining droplet diameters and indicates that, as far as the microdroplets themselves are concerned, the viscosity they experience is that of the continuous phase.

Conductivity of Ionic Microemulsions

There has been little reported work concerning the conductivity of O/W microemulsions stabilized by ionic surfactants. We present here a simple treatment of the conductivity of O/W ionic microemulsions containing no added salt. From this model we calculate the fraction of free counterion (α) and show that a reasonable value, in accord with other measurements, is obtained. We consider the microemulsion to be a 1:q electrolyte, where the charge q on the "droplet

ion" is given by z_2 where z_2 is the total number of surfactant molecules in the drop. The equivalent conductance Λ, based upon the
measured specific conductivity and the total surfactant concentration
in the microemulsion, is then given by

$$\Lambda = (\lambda_1 + \lambda_2)\alpha \qquad \qquad \text{(iv)}$$

where λ_1 and λ_2 are the equivalent conductances of the free counterion
and droplet, respectively. Although a 1mM solution of high-valent
electrolyte is even outside the scope of the Debye-Huckel treatment,
we will use the infinite dilution value of λ_1. The justification for
this simplification is the effective value of lcp for the droplets
(vide supra), the reasonable values obtained, and the current uncer-
taintly in the parameters employed. Then $\lambda_2 = \alpha z_2 D_2 F^2 / RT$, where D_2
is the diffusion coefficient of the drop, and F, R and T are the
Faraday, Gas constant, and absolute temperature, respectively.
Inserting this relation into eq. (iv) and rearranging, we obtain
equation (v),

$$\frac{F^2}{RT} \alpha^2 + \frac{\lambda_1}{z_2 D_2} \alpha - \frac{\Lambda}{z_2 D_2} = 0 \qquad \qquad \text{(v)}$$

The value of z_2 may be obtained from the drop radius (r), which may
be independently determined or calculated from D_2.

Measured values of Λ in the SCS microemulsion along the 21% oil
(initial) dilution line are plotted in Fig. 7, and the values of α
calculated from eq. (v) are shown in Fig. 8. The fraction of free
counterion increases smoothly from about 8% at $\phi = .7$ to 25% at
$\phi = .2$. It is also possible to estimate α from data which relates to
the effective surface potential (ψ) of the microdroplet. Based on a
flat plate model, equation (vi) may be derived[12].

$$\alpha = 2 \left[\frac{4\pi r^2}{e z_2} \right]^2 c \varepsilon N_o kT \left[\exp(\frac{e\psi}{kT}) - 1 \right] \qquad \qquad \text{(vi)}$$

Here, c is the concentration of surfactant, e the electronic charge,
N_o Avogadro's number, k Boltman's constant, and ε the dielectric
constant of the continuous phase (water). From pK measurements in
the $\phi = 0.4$ SCS microemulsion, a potential of 51mV is obtained[7].
From eq. (vi), $\alpha = 0.23$, which may be compared with a value of 0.20
from the conductivity data (Fig. 8).

Microemulsion Viscosities

Thus far, we have employed two "viscosities" in our treatment of
O/W microemulsions. The first one is an effective viscosity experi-

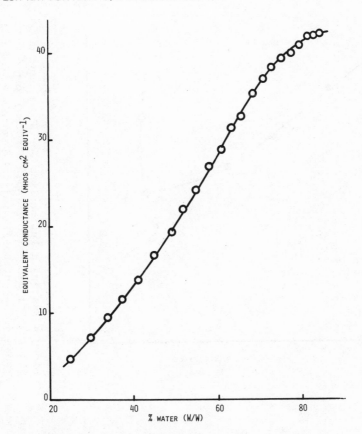

Fig. 7.   Equivalent conductance (Λ) of a SCS/1-pentanol/mineral oil
(21% initial) <u>vs</u> water content.

enced by aqueous ions in their travels through the medium. This
viscosity, $\eta_{eff} = \eta_o(1-\phi)^{-(n+1)}$, where η_o is the continuous phase
viscosity, is related to the "obstruction effect"[6]. The second
viscosity is that experienced by the (ionic) drops, and is apparently
simply η_o. There is of course also a third viscosity, the bulk
viscosity of the microemulsion as determined from a macroscopic
measurement. The relative viscosity (η_r) along a dilution line for
both the Tween 40 and SCS microemulsion is shown in Fig. 9. This
viscosity only plays a role in the hydrodynamic flow of the fluid,
such as in the mass transport of an electroactive species to a rotating platinum electrode. The different viscosities may be a result
of the different size relationships between the species present in
the microemulsion. The aqueous ions are small compared with the drops.
The drops on the other hand are large compared with the solvent molecules, but may be small compared with structures (possibly transient
ones) which determine the bulk viscosity. For example values of D

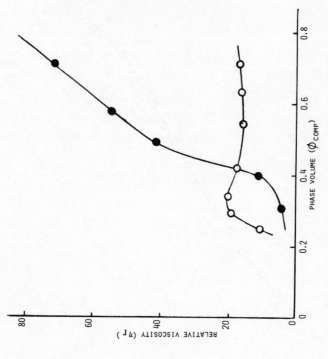

Fig. 9. Relative viscosity vs phase volume along a (water) dilution line for SCS/1-pentanol/21% initial mineral oil (open circles) and Tween 40/1-pentanol/7% initial hexadecane (closed circles) at 25°C.

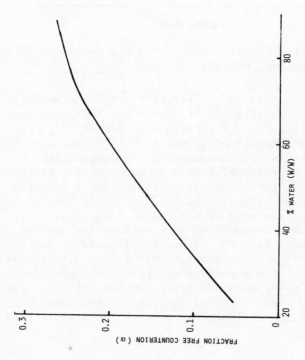

Fig. 8. Fraction of free counterion (α) vs weight % water calculated from conductivity measurements (Figure 6) and equation (v) using $D_{22} = 4 \times 10^{-7}$ cm^{2}s^{-1} $z_2 = 300$ and $\lambda_1 = 50.1$ mho cm^2 equiv^{-1} (Na$^+$).

measured in a nonionic O/W microemulsion using the 1-dodecyl-4-cyano-pyridinium ion exhibits "percolation" type behaviour[13] in that D is low at high water content and increases with decreasing water content. Dynamic clusters resulting from "sticky" collisions between droplets could be responsible for both this and the bulk viscosity.

Summary   We have confirmed the identity of the exponent n in the semi-empirical expressions for the conductance, $\Lambda = \Lambda_o (1-a\phi_{comp})^n$, and diffusion, $D = D_o (1 - \phi_{comp})^{n+1}$, of aqueous ions in nonionic microemulsions. In addition, aqueous ions which are not strongly bound also obey the diffusion equation in ionic microemulsions. Water insoluble electroactive species appear to yield droplet diffusion coefficients in ionic microemulsions which behave as simple 1:q electrolytes. The fraction of free counterion increases with increasing water content to a maximum of about 25%. Different effective viscosities apply to the transport of small molecules, droplets and bulk fluid.

ACKNOWLEDGEMENT

The author wishes to express his thanks to Dr Rameshwar Agarwal for his careful performance of many of the electrochemical measurements. The support of the U.S. Army Research Office is also gratefully acknowledged.

REFERENCES

1. See for example C. A. Jones, L. E. Weaner, and R. A Mackay, J. Phys. Chem., 84 1495 (1980); C. Hermansky and R. A. Mackay, "Solution Chemistry of Surfactants, Vol. 2" K. L. Mittal, Ed., Plenum, New York (1979), pp. 723-730; K. Letts and R. A. Mackay, Inorg. Chem., 14, 2993 (1975), and references contained therein.
2. J. Kiwi and M. Gratzel, J. Am. Chem. Soc., 100, 6314 (1978).
3. G. D. Smith, B. B. Garret, S. L. Holt, and R. E. Barden, J. Phys. Chem., 80, 1708 (1976); A. D. James, B. H. Robinson, and N. C. White, J. Colloid Interface Sci., 59, 328 (1977).
4. E. Sjoblom and S. Friberg, J. Colloid Interface Sci., 67, 16 (1978).
5. M. Dvolaitzky, M. Guyot, M. Lagues, J. P. LePesant, R. Ober, C. Santerey and C. Taupin, J. Chem. Phys., 69, 3279 (1978).
6. R. A. Mackay and R. Agarwal, J. Colloid Interface Sci., 65, 225 (1978).
7. R. A. Mackay, K. Jacobson, and J. Tourian, J. Colloid Interface Sci., 76, 515 (1980).
8. R. A. Mackay, K. Letts and C. Jones, "Micellization, Solubilization, and Microemulsions, Vol. 2", K. L. Mittal, Ed. Plenum, New York (1977), pp. 801-815.
9. C. Hermansky and R. A. Mackay, J. Colloid Interface Sci., 73 324 (1980).

10. R. A. Mackay, C. Hermansky and R. Agarwal, "Colloid and Interface
     Science, Vol. II" M. Kerker, Ed., Academic Press (1976), pp. 289-
     303.
11. J. Novodoff, Henri L. Rosano and H. W. Hoyer, J. Colloid Inter-
     face Sci., 38, 424 (1972).
12. C. Hermansky, Ph.D. Dissertation, Drexel University, Philadelphia
     PA, June 1980.
13. M. Clausse, C. Boned, C. G. Essex, B. Lagourette, V.E.R. McClean,
     J. Peyrelasse and R. J. Sheppard, paper presented at the
     Symposium on Surface Phenomena in Enhanced Oil Recovery,
     Stockholm Sweden, 1979.

DISCUSSION

Mr J. D. Nicholson: Is the Stokes-Einstein equation considered
justifiable to obtain hydrodynamic radius from measured diffusion
coefficients when the microscopic solution viscosities differs from
the solvent. The Stokes-Einstein equation applies strictly only in
the infinite dilution limit for non-interacting spherical particles.

Prof. R. A. Mackay: It is certainly true that the Stokes-Einstein
equation applies strictly only in the infinite dilution limit for
non-interacting particles. However, the conductivity of the ionic
microemulsions appears to be reasonably well described by considering
it to be a simple electrolyte at infinite dilution. The principal
justification at the moment, however, is simply that it appears to
give the correct hydrodynamic radius.

Prof. M. Kahlweit: Is the radius calculated from the diffusion
coefficients independent of composition?

Prof. R. A. Mackay: Yes, it is independent of composition.

Prof. H. T. Davis: (i) It is not surprising that diffusion in a
microemulsion system does not correlate with bulk viscosity. If the
diffusing object is small compared to the length scale of the microstructure controlling bulk viscosity, then the controlling viscosity
is that of local fluid channels contained in the microstructure.
Consider, for example, diffusion of ions in dilute aqueous gel. The
gel can have quite high viscosity while the diffusivities of an ion
are nearly equal to that of the ion in aqueous solution in the absence
of the gelling agent. Actually, since you can determine drop size
independently, comparison of drop diffusion and bulk viscosity
provides an indirect method for putting a lower bound on the characteristic length scale of the microstructure of microemulsion.
(ii) From percolation models of conduction or diffusion in composites
it appears that the conductivity or diffusivity versus volume fraction of a random composite is characterised by two exponents - one
for volume fractions very near the percolation threshold and another
volume fraction away from the threshold. Perhaps your exponent n

would vary less if this concept of two volume fraction domains were introduced.

Prof. R. A. Mackay: (i)   I most certainly agree that the different viscosities must reflect different "structural length" scales with respect to the different moieties being transported.
(ii)   The percolation behaviour should apply to species in the disperse rather than the continuous phase.   Therefore, your suggestion would apply to the diffusion of a water insoluble species in a non-ionic O/W microemulsion, but not to the diffusion of an aqueous ion.

DYNAMIC PROCESSES IN WATER-IN-OIL MICROEMULSIONS

P. D. I. Fletcher, B. H. Robinson, F. Bermejo-Barrera
and D. G. Oakenfull
Chemical Lab., University of Kent at Canterbury, Kent
J. C. Dore and D. C. Steytler
Physics Lab., University of Kent at Canterbury, Kent

We have studied water-in-oil microemulsions formed by the three-component system, aerosol-OT (AOT), water, and heptane. Aerosol-OT is the sodium salt of a dialkylsulphosuccinate and has been much used in the study of the properties of microemulsions since no co-surfactant is required. The main emphasis of our work is on kinetic studies in micro-emulsions, but in connection with these measurements it is essential to obtain as much information as possible concerning the detailed structure of the microemulsions. To this end, we have recently performed some small-angle neutron scattering (SANS) experiments using the facilities available at Harwell and Grenoble.

(1) NEUTRON SCATTERING STUDIES

Using the contrast-variation method, it is possible to obtain information from separate experiments[1,2] on:-

(a) The Water-Core Size (Using H(Heptane), H(Surfactant), D_2O)
and (b) The Overall Size of the Microemulsion Droplet (Using D (Heptane), H(Surfactant), H_2O).

In this way, it is possible to determine (by difference) the thickness of the surfactant coat region. When the concentration of droplets is high, information can also be obtained on interactions between droplets[3].

Some of our main conclusions on the $AOT/H_2O/Heptane$ system are summarised in Table 1.

We find that for R values <30, r_{water} can be determined to $\pm 1 \overset{o}{A}$ and is proportional to $[H_2O]/[AOT]$, as indicated by simple theoretical

Table 1 [x]

$[H_2O]/[AOT] = R$ $[AOT] = 0.05$ mol dm^{-3}	r_{water} (Å) [a]	r_{total} (Å) [b]	Effective [c] surfactant coat thickness (Å)
10 [Reversed Micelle]	26	33	7
15 [Spherical and	30	36	6
20 [apparently mono-	35	42	7
30 [disperse]	48	–	
40 [Not amenable	(60)		
60 [to straight- forward	(90)		
70 [analysis – see text]	(120)		

[x] All data refer to ~25°C

[a] Radius of water core - determined from H(Heptane), H(Surfactant), D_2O experiments.

[b] Overall size of droplet - determined from D(Heptane), H(Surfactant), H_2O experiments.

[c] Given by $r_{total} - r_{water}$.

considerations[4]. The neutron scattering data can be readily fitted
to the appropriate theoretical treatment for monodisperse, spherical,
isolated spheres. For R values >30, a progressively less-good fit is
obtained, which might be consistent with polydispersity or non-spherical structures or size variation within the limits set by our temperature control device (±1°C). However, in this region we are approach-
ing the microemulsion phase boundary where the dispersion exhibits
some curious and interesting properties, e.g. the electrical conductivity is a very sensitive function of temperature (See paper by
H. F. Eicke), and so other interpretations of our data may be possible.
Therefore the values quoted in Table 1 for r_{water} in the case of R>30
only give an approximate indication of size. However, the results
can be seen to be in reasonable agreement with those obtained by

Zulauf and Eicke[5] in iso-octane using photon-correlation spectro-scopy.

We have also been able to take advantage of the sensitivity of the SANS technique in a study of the effect of change in size of the droplets on dilution with the continuous heptane phase. The size of the droplets is not significantly concentration-dependent for R = 20, over the concentration region $[AOT] = 5 \times 10^{-3} - 2 \times 10^{-1}$ mol dm^{-3}. The influence of added salt on droplet size has also been investigated as shown in Table 2.

It would appear that for relatively low R values, where the droplets are monodisperse and stable, the size of the droplet (which already contains a high concentration of Na$^+$ ions) does not change significantly on further addition of salt. However, at higher R values, microemulsions can be destabilised on addition of salt, so that the size is clearly affected in this case.

(2) KINETICS OF SOLUBILIZATE EXCHANGE

Let us consider a bimolecular chemical reaction [Scheme 1] between two hydrophilic reactants A and B to form a product C with all reacting species confined within the dispersed aqueous phase of a microemulsion system, i.e.

$$A \quad + \quad B \quad \longrightarrow \quad C \quad + \quad \bigcirc \quad \ldots (1)$$

Table 2

Effect of Added Salt on Droplet Size.

$[H_2O]/[AOT] = 20$; $[AOT] = 0.05$ mol dm^{-3}

Temperature $= 25\,^{\circ}$C

[salt] [a]	r_{water} (Å)
0	35
0.2 mol dm^{-3} NaNO$_3$	36
0.1 mol dm^{-3} Ni(NO$_3$)$_2$	36
0.05 mol dm^{-3} La(NO$_3$)$_3$	35

[a] Concentration of salt expressed as concentration in water

How does A find B? Does this occur (i) by partition of a reactant molecule out of the water pool, migration through the hydrocarbon
phase and re-entry into a pool containing the other reactant, or (ii)
by direct transfer between pools during the time of the collision
between two droplets. [It should be realised that collisions between
w/o micro-emulsion droplets are much more favourable than collisions
between charged micelles in aqueous solutions.] The possibility of
this process occurring would be enhanced in the case of the more energetic collisions and if collisions were 'sticky'.

Considering the mechanism, Eicke[6] has already shown, using a
hydrophilic fluorescer/quencher system, that inter-droplet communication can be very rapid, and occurs via a transitory 'dimer' species,
formed as a result of droplet collision. Similar conclusions have
been drawn from a study of the Ni^{2+} (aq)/Murexide reaction in the AOT/
H_2O/Heptane system[7], in that exchange of reactants was rapid compared with the time of water exchange at the Ni^{2+} (aq) ion (~1 ms).

However, when the chemical reaction is very fast (as in the case
of many proton/electron transfer reactions or metal-complex formation
involving labile metal ions such as Zn^{2+} (aq), the rate-determining
step in the overall reaction will be the initial communication step
as shown in Scheme 2.

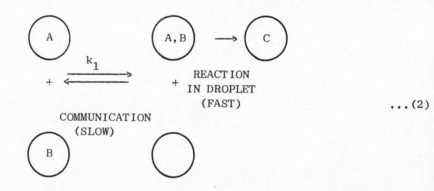

...(2)

The rate of communication may be defined by a second-order comm-
unication-controlled rate constant k_1, expressed in terms of the droplet concentration in heptane and measured in units of dm^3 mol^{-1} s^{-1}.
This rate constant is then analogous to a diffusion-controlled rate
constant in a homogeneous medium, and represents the fastest possible
rate constant for the system. The subsequent reaction (which is not
rate-determining) then simply serves as an indicator that A and B have
communicated, and so in this type of experiment we are basically
monitoring the redistribution of solubilizate molecules between pools.

The kinetics of the following indicator reactions have been
studies by means of the stopped-flow technique with optical detection:

(1)   Proton Transfer:

(2)   Metal-ligand Substitution:

In the experiments, a microemulsion solution containing either solu-bilised H^+ or Zn^{2+} (aq) ions was mixed with a microemulsion containing $NPSA^{2-}$ or Mu^- as appropriate. All reactants partition strongly into the dispersed water phase.

When communication is rate limiting, it is necessary to allow for multiple occupancy of reactants in the pools and to consider both reacting and non-reacting exchange processes[8]. However, all these processes will have the same second-order rate constant after adjust-ment by readily-calculated statistical weighting factors. A large num-ber of related bimolecular steps are therefore involved in the overall reaction (but controlled by a single master rate constant) and so the experimental results were fitted using a large numerical integration program to obtain rate constant k_1.   (Scheme 2)

To test scheme 2 and the general validity of the approach, the following parameters of the system were changed:

  (i)   The numbers of A and B per water pool.
 (ii)   The total droplet concentrations.
(iii)   The Indicator Reaction.
 (iv)   Droplet Size (through variation of R).
  (v)   Temperature.

The mechanism proposed, together with a single value of k_1, could properly represent all kinetic data obtained by variation of para-meters (i) - (iii) to within a self-consistency error of less than 10%, so that k_1 was independent of the reaction chosen for study. (As is also the case for a diffusion-controlled reaction in a homogeneous medium.) A selection of kinetic results is given in Table 3.

Table 3

Variation of k_1 with temperature and R

Temp. (°C)	R = $[H_2O]/[AOT]$	$k_1/dm^3\ mol^{-1}\ s^{-1}$	$\Delta H_1^{\ddagger}/kJ\ mol^{-1}$
10	10	4×10^6	60
20	10	1×10^7	
10	15	3×10^6	77
20	15	7.5×10^6	
10	20	2×10^6	89
20	20	6×10^6	

The results may be summarised as follows:

k_1 is $\sim 10^6$-10^7 $dm^3\ mol^{-1}\ s^{-1}$. Hence we can conclude that approximately 1 in 10^3 of the collisions between droplets leads to exchange, since k_D is $\sim 10^{10}$ $dm^3\ mol^{-1}\ s^{-1}$ in a solvent with the viscosity of n-heptane. These values also imply that at a droplet concentration of $>10^{-3}$ $mol\ dm^{-3}$, exchange will be effectively complete within 1 ms. It is, however, clear that exchange does not take place very often; presumably only the more energetic collisions are able to establish a water channel since the activation energy of the process ($\Delta H_1^{\ddagger}$) is much greater than that corresponding to a diffusion or entropy-controlled process. The interaction between w/o microemulsion droplets is generally considered as being of the hard-sphere type with a small attractive term. This is consistent with the picture emerging from the kinetic studies.

Our results also indicate that exchange becomes slightly more difficult as the droplet size increases in the 20-30 Å region.

These results have some important general implications for kinetic studies in microemulsion systems, if we can safely generalise from our initial results using the AOT system. They are:

(a) For reactions on the nsec time scale (e.g. fluorescence quenching studies) droplets are essentially isolated and 'frozen'.

(b) For reaction processes in the μsec to msec time range, the communication process is rate-limiting and reactant concentration in discrete pools must be considered in any kinetic analysis. (Also in (a)).

(c) For reactions occurring in longer times, the disperse water phase

can be effectively regarded as 'continuous' since communication is
not rate-limiting. This simplifies the kinetics considerably[7] since
only the overall concentration of reactants in the water phase need be
considered.

(d) For these 'slow' reactions, we obtain no information on the kinetics and mechanism of communication since it is not rate-limiting, but
we are able to investigate how the dispersed water and confinement
within a droplet can influence the reaction as compared with a bulk
water environment. The kinetics of a 'slow' reaction will now be considered to demonstrate this approach.

(3) THE REACTION BETWEEN Ni^{2+} (aq) AND MUREXIDE IN MICROEMULSION/
     REVERSED MICELLE WATER POOLS

Let us consider whether we can obtain dramatic promotion/inhibi-
tion effects for metal-ligand substitution reactions in microemulsions
as has been onserved previously[9,10] in aqueous micellar systems.

The reaction scheme is now as shown in (3)

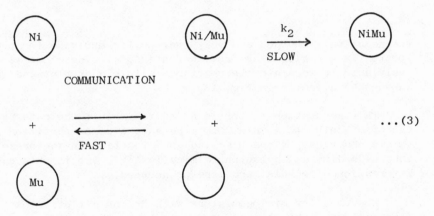

The rate constant k_2 is made up of the product of a fast pre-
equilibrium term describing the distribution/location of the reactants
within a water-pool prior to reaction and a first-order rate constant
k_{WE} which corresponds to the process of removal of a water molecule
from the metal ion prior to ligand binding. [A 'dissociative' mechanism operates for this reaction in an aqueous medium].

These two factors, which can influence the reaction rate in w/o
microemulsions, (stabilized by charged surfactants), will now be considered in more detail.

(a) REACTANT PARTITIONING INSIDE A WATER DROPLET

Because the AOT interface is negatively charged, the Ni^{2+} (aq)
ion will be preferentially located close to this interface, whereas

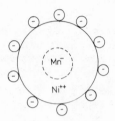

Fig.1.   Location of Ni^{2+} (aq) and Mu^- within a medium-sized pool
(e.g. R ∼20).

the negatively-charged and very hydrophilic murexide ion prefers to be
located in a region away from the interface.   Therefore we are effectively able to separate the reactants within a droplet, and this is
shown schematically in Fig. 1.

     This separation factor is found to inhibit the rate by a maximum
factor of only ∼10 at R = 20.   (The same type of partitioning behaviour is observed for the Ni^{2+} (aq)/Mu^- reaction in the presence of
aqueous sodium dodecylsulphate micelles[10], but in this case the
retardation effect is much more pronounced.).

     However, for microemulsions with R<5 no effective partitioning
(separation) within a pool can occur since the pools are very small
and hence no retardation due to this effect is possible.   Also, for
very large pools, the surface/volume ratio is reduced, and partitioning due to this effect (and the rate inhibition) should be again less
pronounced.

(b)   THE WATER-EXCHANGE RATE AT THE NICKEL ION

     For the Ni^{2+}/Mu^- reaction in bulk water, the rate-determining
step is loss of water from the metal ion which is identified with the
water-exchange rate as measured by nmr methods.   This process can also
be shown to be rate-limiting in the microemulsion/reversed-micelle
systems we have investigated.   Fortunately, in the microemulsion system, it is possible to determine this rate constant (k_{WE}) directly
from our kinetic measurements (which were again obtained using the

Table 4

Variation of k_{WE} with water-pool size*

Temperature = $25^{\circ}C$

No. of water molecules/pool	R	k_{WE}/s^{-1}
∞	∞	$\sim10^4$
	(bulk water)	
2000	13	9×10^3
400	6	$>1 \times 10^3$
300	4.6	70
220	3.7	60
150	2.8	70

stopped-flow technique with optical detection. Details will be given in a full paper[11].

Values of k_{WE} as a function of water-pool size (expressed as number of water molecules per pool) are given in Table 4.

*

We may conclude that for R< 6, [i.e. when there are less than 6 water molecules for each Na^+ ion in the pool], all the water molecules in the pool are effectively involved in solvation. In this situation we observe a sharp reduction in rate (from Table 4) as the water molecules are then apparently more tightly bound to the Ni^{2+} ion, inhibiting ligand substitution by Mu^-. However, the overall effects are not particularly pronounced and it is reasonable to conclude that even the water in the smallest pools studied is quite similar to bulk water as far as it functions as an aqueous reaction medium. Similar conclusions have recently been reached from the study of enzyme reactions in microemulsions[12]. Therefore we may conclude, in the absence of the surfactant acting as a type of 'functional' reversed micelle, that microemulsions will generally influence the rates of reactions involving metal ions to a lesser extent than charged micelles in aqueous solution.

ACKNOWLEDGEMENTS

We thank the S.R.C. for financial support in connection with equipment and facilities used in this work.

REFERENCES

1. M. Dvolaitzky, M. Guyot, M. Lagües, J. P. Le Pasant, R. Ober,
    C. Sauterey and C. Taupin, J. Chem. Phys., 69, 3279 (1978).
2. C. Cabos and P. DeLord, J. Appl. Cryst., 12, 502, (1979).
3. D. J. Cebula, L. Harding, R. H. Ottewill and P. N. Pusey, Colloid
    and Polymer Science, (1980). In press.
4. D. G. Oakenfull, J. Chem. Soc. Faraday Trans. 1, 76, 1875 (1980)
5. M. Zulauf and H. F. Eicke, J. Phys. Chem., 83 480, (1979).
6. H. F. Eicke, J. C. W. Shepherd and A. Steinemann, J. Colloid
    Interface Sci., 56, 168, (1976).
7. B. H. Robinson, D. C. Steytler and R. D. Tack, J. Chem. Soc.
    Faraday Trans. 1, 75 781, (1979).
8. P. D. I. Fletcher and B. H. Robinson, to be published.
9. A. D. James and B. H. Robinson, J. Chem. Soc. Faraday Trans. 1,
    74, 10, (1978).
10. M. Fischer, W. Knoche, P. D. I. Fletcher and B. H. Robinson,
    Colloid and Polymer Science, 258, 733, (1980).
11. D. G. Oakenfull and B. H. Robinson, to be published.
12. F. M. Menger and K. Yamada, J. Amer. Chem. Soc., 101, 6731, (1979

Dr I. D. Robb: What is the state of the dimers in the 'sticky collision' that allows transfer but no long term coagulation?

Dr B. H. Robinson: From our kinetic results we can only infer that
reactants are transferred into the same pool in approximately 1 in
10^3 of the collisions between droplets. This does not necessarily
imply a 'sticky' collision but neither can the collision process be
totally elastic.

We can represent the process of association of droplets by the
following series of equilibria:

$$\text{Mon} + \text{Mon} \xrightleftharpoons{k_1} \text{Dimer}$$

$$\text{Dimer} + \text{Mon} \xrightleftharpoons{k_2} \text{Trimer}$$

$$n\text{Mer} + \text{Mon} \xrightleftharpoons{k_n} (n + 1) \text{Mer}$$

$$K_n = \frac{k_n}{k_{-n}}$$

Since there seems to be no reason to invoke positive cooperativity in the aggregation process (as is found in micellar association),
we can suppose that $K_1 > K_n$. (As is observed for the association of
planar dyes in aqueous solution).

Then, provided that the 'lifetime" of the dimer formed on collision is less than the time required for another droplet to find the dimer and associate to form the trimer (i.e. $k_{-1} > k_2 [\text{Mon}]$), no significant build up of aggregates can occur so that coalescence is prevented. We would suppose the lifetime of the dimer to be less than 1 µs so the condition is easily fulfilled.

A consequence of this approach is that the equilibrium concentration of dimers (and higher aggregates) should increase with the total concentration of droplets, and it might be possible to observe such species using modern physical methods.

Prof J. Th. G. Overbeek: When you talk about sticky collisions you seem to imply that about 1 in 1000 collisions is of such a nature that a water channel is opened up. Could it not be that all collisions are of the same nature with a water channel opening for a very short time and that only in 1 in 1000 cases the Ni^{2+} ion or other reactant succeeds in passing through the channel?

Dr B. H. Robinson: From our kinetic measurements so far, it is difficult to draw conclusions on the precise mechanism of transfer.

The process may occur as suggested above, but we have found the exchange process to be associated with a relatively high activation energy (Table 3) which tends to suggest that only the more energetic collisions can generate a water channel. Once a water channel is formed diffusion into the other pool should be a very rapid process. Alternatively, it may be that reactants diffuse between the surfactant chains in the dimer.

ULTRASONIC RELAXATION STUDIES OF MICROEMULSIONS

J. Lang, A. Djavanbakht and R. Zana

CNRS, Centre de Recherches sur les Macromolecules
6, rue Boussingault
67083 Strasbourg-Cedex - France

INTRODUCTION

The main purpose of the ultrasonic absorption studies of micro-emulsions reported in this paper, as well as in a previous one[1] (referred to as Part I in the following) was to reach a better under-standing of the dynamic properties of microemulsions. Indeed, it has been put forward[2] that these properties may play an important role in determining the stability of microemulsions.

In Part I, two types of ultrasonic absorption studies were performed on microemulsions. First, we compared the ultrasonic absorption of microemulsions with compositions close to a demixing curve or corresponding to a transition region of the phase diagrams to the absorption of binary systems where concentration fluctuations were known to occur. Ternary systems were also studied. The microemulsions were made of water/sodium dodecylsulfate (SDS)/1-pentanol/cyclohexane with a weight ratio (water)/(SDS) = 2.5, and water/SDS/1-butanol/ toluene with a weight ratio (butanol)/(SDS) = 2 (these two systems will be referred to as Systems I and IIa respectively throughout this paper). The results led us to conclude that the critical character (fluctuations) of a system becomes less and less marked as the number of components in the system is increased[1]. Note however that the experiments performed at a frequency of 2.8MHz on System I showed the existence of a maximum of absorption at a composition corresponding closely to that where electrical conductivity and neutron scatter-ing[3,4] indicate a transition from an oil-in-water (O/W) type micro-emulsion, to a water-in-oil (W/O) type microemulsion. No maximum was observed with System IIa.

The second type of experiments concerned the ultrasonic relaxa-

tion behaviour of microemulsions from the System IIa. For five out
of the seven investigated microemulsions the results showed the existence of two fast ultrasonic relaxation processes which were attributed to the exchange of the surfactant and alcohol between the microemulsion interfacial film and the continuous aqueous phase by analogy
with the results obtained with the ternary systems water/surfactant/
alcohol[5]. A single relaxation process was observed with a microemulsion where the continuous phase was believed to be essentially
made of toluene. This preliminary result suggested the possibility
of monitoring the W/O to O/W microemulsion transition by means of the
ultrasonic absorption.

     In the present work we have greatly extended our ultrasonic
relaxation investigations of microemulsions by determining the ultrasonic relaxation spectra of

   (i)   seven microemulsions of System I,
  (ii)   twelve additional microemulsions of System IIa, in order to
         complete the study of this system,
 (iii)   eight microemulsions of System III: water/SDS/1-pentanol/
         dodecane, with a weight ratio (pentanol)/(SDS) = 2.

     We have also measured the change of the ultrasonic absorption
at a given frequency with composition for a series of microemulsions
of the System IIb: water/SDS/1-butanol/toluene with a weight ratio
(water)/(SDS) = 2.58.

     The purpose of these various experiments was to have a suffi-
ciently large number of data in order to

   (i) compare the ultrasonic absorption and relaxation behaviour of
systems where the ratio (alcohol)/(SDS) remains constant to that of
systems where the ratio (water)/(SDS) is kept constant,

  (ii) determine the number of ultrasonic relaxation processes which
characterize microemulsions for a large number of compositions and
for several systems in order to attribute more safely these processes
and to study them, in particular for compositions in the range where
the W/O to O/W transition occurs.

EXPERIMENTAL SECTION

     The SDS sample used in these studies was purchased from Touzart
and Matignon. Its CMC as determined by means of electrical conductivity was found to be $(8.5 \pm 0.2) \times 10^{-3}M$ in excellent agreement with
the literature value, and was negligibly affected by recrystalliza-
tion in water-alcohol mixtures. The SDS was therefore used without
further purification throughout this work.

     Toluene, cyclohexane, 1-butanol and 1-pentanol were the same as in Part I. Dodecane (purity 99%) was obtained from Aldrich.

For the various investigated Systems (I, IIa, IIb and III) the microemulsions with compositions falling close to a demixing line were prepared as previously described[1]. Other compositions were prepared by simply weighing the various constituents. All the investigated solutions were stable, transparent and macroscopically homogeneous.

The ultrasonic absorption α/f^2 (α = absorption coefficient in cm^{-1}, f = frequency in Hz) were measured in the frequency range 1.04 to 156 MHz by means of the same equipment as in Part I. The ultrasonic relaxation spectra (α/f^2 vs f plots) were fitted to the relaxation equation with two relaxation terms:

$$\frac{\alpha}{f^2} \simeq \frac{A_1}{1+(f/f_{R1})^2} + \frac{A_2}{1+(f/f_{R2})^2} + B \qquad \ldots(1)$$

where B is a constant, A_1 and A_2 the relaxation amplitudes and f_{R1} and f_{R2} the relaxation frequencies which are related to the relaxation times τ by : $\tau_{1,2} = (2\pi f_{R1,2})^{-1}$. The quantities A_1, A_2, f_{R1}, f_{R2} and B were obtained by a weighted least-square procedure[6]. For three of the investigated systems, the relaxation spectra could be fitted to equation 1 with A_1 or A_2 = 0.

RESULTS

System I. The ultrasonic relaxation spectra of the solutions corresponding to the representative points S28 to S34 along the demixing line on the phase diagram of this System (see Fig. 1) have been determined. A typical relaxation spectrum is given in Fig. 2, where curve 1 corresponds to a fitting of the data to equation 1 (two relaxation terms) and curve 2 to a fitting of the data to equation 1 with A_2=0 (one relaxation term). This example clearly shows that the full equation 1 gives a much better fit to the data.

The values of A_1, A_2, f_{R1}, f_{R2} and B for the investigated solutions are listed in Table I. The variations of f_{R1} and f_{R2}, and A_1 and A_2 are represented as a function of the water volume fraction ψ_w in Fig. 3 and 4, respectively. At around ψ_w = 0.33, where other studies[4] indicate that O/W microemulsions turn into W/O microemulsions, both relaxation amplitudes go through a marked maximum whereas the associated relaxation frequencies go through a minimum. The results of Fig. 3 and 4 confirm our previous observation[1] that the ultrasonic absorption at 2.8 MHz goes through a maximum at about the same value of ψ_w.

System IIa. The ultrasonic relaxation spectra of the solutions

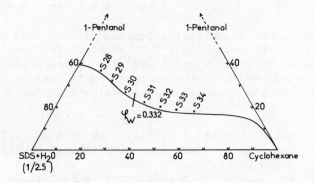

Fig. 1.   Phase diagram of the water/SDS/1-pentanol/cyclohexane:
System I at 25°C.   The W/O to O/W transition occurs at ψ_w = 0.332 on
the demixing line.

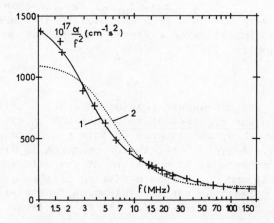

Fig. 2.   Relaxation spectrum of solution S29 at 25°C.   (+) :
Experimental results.   (———): Fitting to the full equation 1.
(....) :   Fitting to the equation 1 with A_2=0.

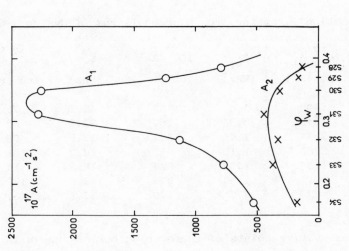

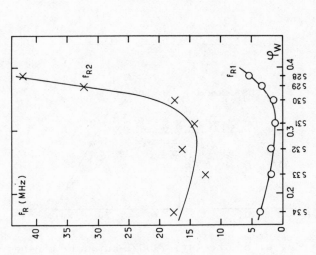

Fig. 4. Variation of the relaxation amplitudes for the solutions S28 to S34 for System I, with the water volume fraction ψ_w at 25°C.

Fig. 3. Variation of the relaxation frequencies of the solutions S28 to S34 for System I, with the water volume fraction ψ_w at 25°C.

Table 1:   Relaxation Parameters for Microemulsions of System I at 25°C

Micro emulsion[a]	$10^{17} A_1$ $(cm^{-1}s^2)$	f_{R1} (MHz)	$10^{17} A_2$ $(cm^{-1} s^2)$	f_{R2} (MHz)	$10^{17} B$ $(cm^{-1}s^2)$
S28	792	5.4	132	42.1	75
S29	1243	3.3	167	32.2	83
S30	2264	1.45	317	17.5	90
S31	2286	1.13	411	14.2	101
S32	1134	1.84	334	16.3	114
S33	771	1.94	374	12.5	137
S34	529	3.7	179	17.8	161

(a)   The representative points of these solutions are shown in Fig. 1.

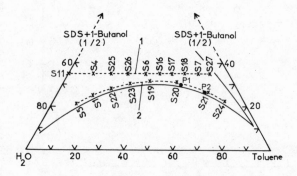

Fig. 5.   Phase diagram of the water/SDS/1-butanol/toluene: System IIa at 20°C as reported by ARTEP (see Part I) and in reference 18.

Table II: Relaxation parameters for microemulsions of System IIa at $25\,^{\circ}C$

Micro-emulsion[a]	$10^{17}\,A_1$ $(cm^{-1}s^2)$	f_{R1} (MHz)	$10^{17}\,A_2$ $(cm^{-1}s^2)$	f_{R2} (MHz)	$10^{17}\,B$ $(cm^{-1}s^2)$
S1[b]	1342	2.6	528	23.3	79
S4[b]	783	6.4	252	43.2	72
S5[b]	1322	2.75	716	22	55
S6[b]	546	4.5	141	33.5	79
S7[c]	32	7	42	32	76
S7[b]	63.6	19.3			78
S11[b]	466	19.3	162	82	73
S16	438	4.2	106	38.1	76
S17	295	4.5	87	33.7	77
S18	152	5.5	57	31.3	79
S19	558	3.3	173	27.9	87
S20	397	2.9	98	26.8	90
S21	156	5.3	27.4	49.7	86
S22	793	3.8	325	29.2	76
S23	715	3.5	234	37.4	65
S24[c]	130	6.0	26	45	93
S24	114	9.8			99
S25	766	4.8	233	36.8	72
S26	692	4.4	183	39.3	70
S27			43.3	24.7	76

(a) The representative points for the various solutions are shown on Figure 5.
(b) Data from ref. 1.
(c) Values obtained as described in the text.

corresponding to the representative points S16 to S27 on the phase diagram of System IIa (see Fig. 5) have been determined. As can be seen on Fig. 5 the representative points of these solutions and those investigated in Part I from the same System define two lines : line 1 which corresponds to experiments where the percentage of active mixture SDS + butanol remains constant and line 2 which closely follows the demixing line. The relaxation parameters for the various spectra

are given in Table II. The variations of the relaxation frequencies
and amplitudes for the two series of experiments are shown in Figures
6 to 9. As can be seen in Table II the results for the compositions
S7, S24 and S27 could be fitted to a single relaxation term equation.
No convergence of the least square calculation could be obtained with
the full equation 1. This however is mainly due to the small magnitude of the relaxation amplitude for these three systems. Indeed,
calculations showed that the spectra S7 and S24 could be equally well
fitted with the full equation 1, when the values of the five relaxation parameters were obtained by extrapolating the curves representing
the variations of the relaxation parameters for the other investigated
solutions, with composition. In the case of composition S27 the
extrapolated value of A_1 was zero. However the results plotted on
Fig. 6 and 7 show that the values of the relaxation frequency and
amplitude obtained from the fit of the S27 relaxation spectra to
equation 1 with A_1=0 fall nicely on the A_2 and f_{R2} vs toluene weight
percent curves. In Part I, S7 was fitted to a single relaxation
frequency equation and the question was raised on whether one would
not go from two to one relaxation process in going from O/W to W/O
microemulsions, as S7 was believed to be in the W/O range and the
other solutions in the O/W range. In view of the present results this
does not seem to be the case and all the microemulsions of System I
and IIa, but S27 for the reason given above, whether close or far from
the demixing line appear to be characterized by two relaxation processes.

For the solutions along line 1 in Fig. 5 the relaxation frequencies first decrease and then remain practically constant, whereas both
relaxation amplitudes go through a maximum as the toluene content is
increased (Fig. 6 and 7). The solutions along the demixing line showed
a slightly different behaviour in that the relaxation amplitudes
decrease and the relaxation frequencies increase slightly as the toluene content is increased (Fig. 8 and 9). Thus the behaviour of the
relaxation amplitudes of System IIa differs strongly from that of
System I.

System IIb. This System differs from System IIa in that the
(water)/(SDS) ratio, rather than the (butanol)/(SDS) ratio, is kept
constant. The phase diagram is shown in Fig. 10. The absorption measurements were performed at 2.8MHz, as a function of composition
(water volume fraction) along the demixing line and the results are
shown on Fig. 11. A maximum of small amplitude is observed for a
water volume fraction ψ_w = 0.42. Electrical conductivity measurements performed on the same System reveal a change of slope at about
the same ψ_w [7] which is very likely associated with the W/O to O/W
inversion, by analogy with the results for the System I. Thus for the
two Systems I and IIb where the ratio (water)/(SDS) was kept constant,
the ultrasonic absorption vs composition curves present a maximum for
a composition corresponding to the inversion of the microemulsion type.
No such maximum was observed in similar measurements performed with

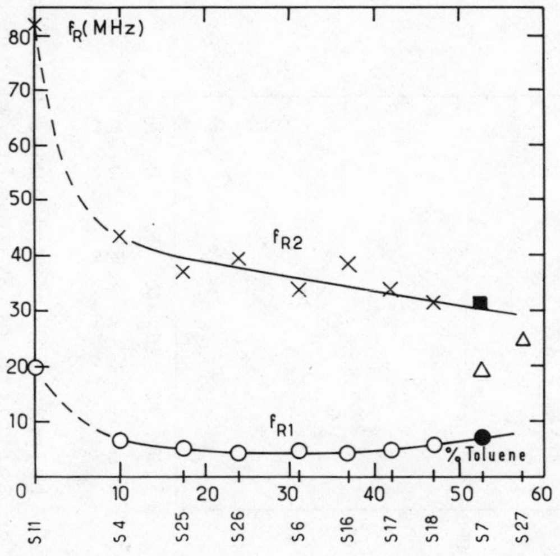

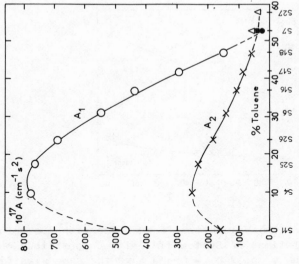

Fig. 7. Variation of the relaxation amplitudes with the toluene weight percent for the solutions of System IIa, with compositions on line 1 at 25°C. Δ, ● and ■ have the same signification as in Figure 6.

Fig. 6. Variation of the relaxation frequencies with the toluene weight percent for the solutions of System IIa, with compositions on line 1 at 25°C. (Δ): Value of f_R for a fitting of the results for S7 to equation 1 with $A_2=0$. (●,■): Values of f_{R1} and f_{R2} for S7, obtained as explained in the text.

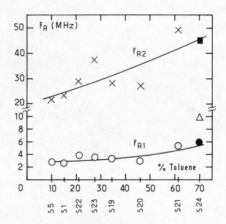

Fig. 8. Variation of the relaxation frequencies with the toluene
content, for the solutions of System IIa, with compositions on line 2
at 25°C. For S24 the symbols Δ, ● and ■ have the same significance
as for S7 in Fig. 6.

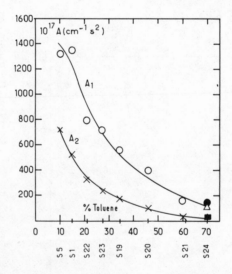

Fig. 9. Variation of the relaxation amplitudes with the toluene
weight percent for the solutions of System Ia, with compositions on
line 2 at 25°C. For S24 the symbols Δ, ● and ■ have the same significance as for S7 in Fig. 6.

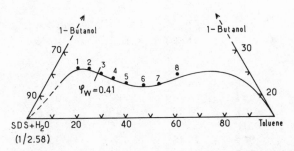

Fig. 10. Phase diagram of the water/SDS/1-butanol/toluene: System IIb at 25°C. The ultrasonic absorption has been measured for compositions 1 to 8 (see Figure 11). The W/O to O/W transition occurs at $\psi_W = 0.41$ on the demixing curve (from reference 7).

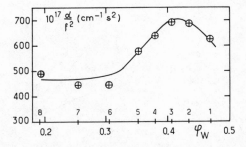

Fig. 11. Variation of the ultrasonic absorption at 2.8MHz and 25°C for solutions of System IIb, with the water volume fraction ψ_w, for compositions close to the demixing curve as shown on Figure 10.

Table III : Relaxation Parameters for Microemulsions of System III
at $20^{\circ}C$

Micro-emulsion (a)	$10^{17} A_1$ (cm^{-1} s^2)	f_{R1} (MHz)	$10^{17} A_2$ (cm^{-1} s^2)	f_{R2} (MHz)	$10^{17} B$ (cm^{-1} s^2)
S35	1668	3.81	460	15.3	60
S36	1584	3.74	397	17.2	76.5
S37	1361	3.26	389	15.7	96.6
S38	1048	2.05	495	12.6	108
S39	954	1.48	434	11.6	113
S40	513	3.48	154	20.3	108
S41	224	6.46	42.6	55	100
S42	68	4.63	28	78	88.3

(a) The representative points of these solutions are shown in
Fig. 10.

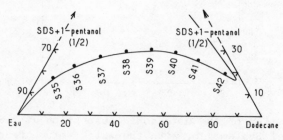

Fig. 12. Phase diagram of the water/SDS/1-pentanol/dodecane:
System III at 20°, from ARTEP (see Part I).

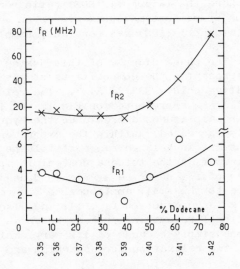

Fig. 13. Variation of the relaxation frequencies with the dodecane weight percent for the solutions of System III at 20°C.

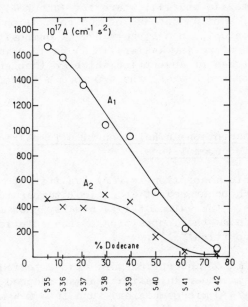

Fig. 14: Variation of the relaxation amplitudes with the dodecane weight percent for the solutions of System III at 20°C.

the System IIa, where the (alcohol)/(SDS) ratio remained constant.
This result led us to perform measurements on an additional system
where the ratio (alcohol)/(SDS) was constant, namely the System III.

System III. The phase diagram of this System is shown on Fig. 12
where are also represented the compositions of the solutions investigated (representative points S35 to S42). The relaxation parameters
listed in Table III are represented on Fig.13 and 14. As for System
IIa, the relaxation amplitudes decrease as the hydrocarbon content
(here, dodecan) is increased. Within the experimental error f_{R2}
remains about constant in a large range of toluene content whereas f_{R1}
goes through a minimum as the toluene content is increased. The
important increase of f_{R2} observed at higher dodecane content may
essentially be due to the small amplitude of the relaxation process
which results in a large error on f_{R2}. It may also reflect the occurrence of an additional relaxation process which is not detected with
the other solutions simply because of its very small amplitude relative to the other two relaxation process which are observed at lower
dodecane content.

Nevertheless the comparison of the four investigated Systems
reveals a clear difference in the behaviour of the ultrasonic absorption. The Systems IIa and III, where the (alcohol)/(SDS) ratio
remains constant, show a decrease of the relaxation amplitudes upon
increasing oil content, in a large range of composition, whereas the
Systems I and IIb where the (water)/(SDS) ratio remains constant have
relaxation amplitudes or absorption which go through a marked maximum
in the composition range where the W/O to O/W transformation occurs.

DISCUSSION

1) Ultrasonic Absorption in Relation with Transitions and Critical
   Phenomena in Microemulsions

The ultrasonic absorption is very sensitive to the concentration
fluctuations which occur near the critical temperature or composition
in binary liquids. The value of α/f^2 usually goes through a maximum
of large amplitude as the composition of the solution is varied around
the critical composition[8-11].

Similar maxima of absorption were also expected as the composition of the systems under investigation was changed in the range of
composition where W/O microemulsions turn into O/W microemulsions,
had long-range composition fluctuations been present in this region.
In that respect, the maxima of A_1 and A_2 in Fig. 4 for System I and
of α/f^2 in Fig. 11 for System IIb may, at first examination, be attributed to composition fluctuations since these maxima occur at water
volume fractions close to those for which other measurements indicate
a transition from W/O to O/W microemulsions for these two systems.
This is not believed to be the case, however, essentially because the

fluctuation theory leads to predict a linear variation of α/f^2 with $f^{-5/4}$, which is not confirmed by all of the spectra relative to System Systems I, IIa and III.

Another fact which goes against the attribution of the maxima of Fig. 4 and 11 to composition fluctuations is the absence of a maximum in the variation of the relaxation amplitudes with composition for the Systems IIa and III, where the (alcohol)/(SDS) weight ratio is kept constant (see Fig. 7, 9 and 14), as the composition is varied in a large range both along the demixing line and far from it. Note that one reaches the water apex of the phase diagram at low toluene (System IIa) and dodecane (System III) contents. Since the absorption of water is very low, the relaxation amplitudes of the solutions are therefore likely to go through a maximum, as the toluene or dodecane content is decreased further in Fig. 9 and 14. These maxima however would only result from the chemical composition of the investigated systems and not from some peculiar effects.

2) Origin of the Ultrasonic Relaxation Processes in Microemulsions

It is well established that the fast exchange of surfactant ions between the micelles and the bulk solution is responsible for the excess ultrasonic absorption of aqueous micellar solutions[12,13]. The relaxation frequency for this process is of about 2 MHz for an 0.1 M SDS solution[1]. This frequency is increased if an additive which is partitioned between the micelles and the bulk, such as an alcohol of medium chain length, is introduced in the micellar solution[1,5]. Besides, this additive gives rise to an additional relaxation process due to its own exchange between the mixed surfactant + additive micelles and the bulk[5]. With medium chain length alcohols (1-butanol to 1-hexanol) this relaxation process is likely to be faster than that for the SDS exchange, in view of the results obtained with other alcohol + surfactant systems[5]. Therefore the ternary water/SDS/alcohol systems should be characterized by two fast exchange processes, the slow process being due to the surfactant exchange and the fast one to the alcohol exchange. In going from these ternary systems to microemulsions by progressive addition of oil, the two exchange processes are going to remain operative even though their characteristics will be modified by the introduction of oil. It is therefore very likely that in water-rich systems, where the continuous phase is water and where the droplets are simply oil swollen micelles, the two observed ultrasonic relaxation processes are due to the alcohol and surfactant exchanges, as in the case of the ternary water/surfactant/alcohol systems. Note however that the exchange is now going to occur between the droplet interfacial layer and the bulk, rather than between the bulk micelle and the bulk solution. It could be argued that in the case of O/W microemulsions the self-association of the alcohol present in the water continuous phase may be responsible for one of the two observed relaxation processes since aqueous solutions of short chain alcohol (linear alcohols up to 1-propanol, and t-butanol) do indeed show a large excess absorption due to such processes[14-16]. However measurements performed as part of this work showed that saturated 1-pentanol aqueous solutions have the same absorption as water, whereas aqueous solutions of 1-butanol show a slight excess absorption with respect to water from a concentration above about 0.85 $\underline{M}$ to the saturation (about 0.97 $\underline{M}$). In view of these results the self-association of the alcohol in the water phase can be discarded as a possible mechanism of absorption in O/W microemulsions, where we are just left with the two exchange processes.

We now examine the results relative to W/O microemulsions, that is systems in the oil-rich part of the phase diagram, and we first restrict ourselves to systems very rich in oil, where the existence of water droplets surrounded by a surfactant + alcohol interfacial layer can reasonably be assumed. Here again the results show the existence of two ultrasonic relaxation processes, the attribution of which is not as easy as in the case of water-rich O/W microemulsions. Indeed these two processes may arise from:

1) the self-association of the alcohol in the oil phase,
2) the exchange of the oil adsorbed in the interfacial film between this film and the bulk oil phase,
3) the exchange of the alcohol and surfactant between the interfacial film on the one hand and the bulk oil phase and/or the water dispersed phase on the other hand.

These various processes will be successively examined.

The self-association of alcohols in organic solvents through H-bonds has been extensively investigated by means of ultrasonic relaxation methods[6]. The oil continuous phase of W/O microemulsions contains alcohol and a small amount of water. Its composition can be obtained by the dilution method[17]. In particular the composition of the continuous phase of microemulsions of System IIa has been determined[18]. Two typical continuous phase compositions represented by the points P1 and P2 in Fig. 5, with the following weight percents of toluene, 1-butanol and water : 76.4, 22.7 and 0.9 for P1 and 83.3, 16 and 0.7 for P2, have been studied. No relaxation process was found for these two solutions. Therefore the alcohol self-association in the oil phase cannot be responsible for the observed relaxations.

The combination of various methods indicates that the interfacial film is solvated up to a certain extent by the oil, which penetrates between the surfactant chains[3]. The exchange of this oil between the adsorbed state and the bulk (free) state is however very unlikely to contribute to the observed relaxation. Indeed such an exchange would give rise to a relaxation excess absorption only if a sizable volume change and/or enthalpy change are associated with this process [19]. This cannot be the case in W/O microemulsions as the absorbed oil remains located fairly far from the polar groups of the inter-solution.

The exchange of the alcohol can occur between the interfacial
film and the oil phase and also between this film and the dispersed
aqueous phase, since the alcohols used in the present study are miscible with toluene and dodecane, and sufficiently soluble in water.
These two exchanges may be then assumed to be responsible for the
observed two relaxation processes. However, this assumption does not
hold when one examines the changes of f_{R1} and f_{R2} with composition for
System I as ψ_w is progressively decreased and the O/W microemulsion
turns into a W/O microemulsion. Indeed, the change of the two relaxation frequencies is very progressive (see Fig. 3). It shows no evidence which would permit one to assume that the slow process, which
is associated to the surfactant exchange in O/W systems, should be
assigned to the alcohol exchange once the O/W to W/O transition region
is passed. It is rather believed that the two exchange equilibria
involving the alcohol occur at comparable rates and, within the experimental uncertainty, are detected as a single relaxation process. This
is clearly the case for O/W systems, and since f_{R2} changes only slowly
with composition it is also probably the case for W/O systems. The
attribution of the fast relaxation process to the alcohol exchange is
supported by the fact that the values of f_{R2} for pentanol-containing
systems are always smaller than for butanol-containing systems. Such
a difference is expected on the basis of the ultrasonic absorption
studies of the water/surfactant/alcohol systems[5].

For the investigated W/O systems, the exchange of the surfactant
can occur only between the interfacial film and the dispersed aqueous
phase since SDS is practically insoluble in toluene, dodecane, butanol
and pentanol. The next question is then to know whether this process
can give rise to a measurable ultrasonic absorption. This appears to
be the case. Indeed the dispersed aqueous phase contains some alcohol
(at a concentration probably lower than the saturation concentration)
and surfactant, at a concentration probably close to the critical
micelle concentration (cmc) in a water-alcohol mixture with the same
alcohol content as the dispersed phase. On the basis of reported
results[20] for SDS in water-alcohol mixtures this cmc is of about
5×10^{-3} M. The radius of the minimum water droplet containing one
surfactant, and such that the surfactant concentration within the
droplet is 5×10^{-3} M is found to be 42 Å, that is a value well within
the range found for microemulsions[21]. For a qualitative comparison
the expression of the amplitude of the ultrasonic relaxation for the
surfactant exchange can then be obtained using a classical procedure[19]. On the assumption of a volume change of 11 cm³/mole for the
transfer of one surfactant from the film to the water core[22,23], one
finds

$$A_1 \approx 10^{-8} \; \psi_w/f_{R1} \qquad\qquad ...(2)$$

This equation correctly predicts the observed decrease of A_1 with decreasing ψ_w. In fact for System IIa where f_{R1} is almost constant in the oil phase (see Fig. 6), equation 2 predicts a linear decrease upon increasing oil volume fraction, as indeed observed. However, the calculated values of A_1 are much smaller than the experimental ones. For instance, with System IIa, A_1 is calculated to be 62×10^{-17} cm^{-1}s^2 for $\psi_w = 0.26$ and $f_{R1} = 4.2$ MHz (from S16 in Fig. 6) whereas the experimental value is 440×10^{-17} cm^{-1}s^2 (see Table II).

One additional remark should be made concerning the slow relaxation: f_{R1} varies only in a fairly narrow range, between 1 and 7 MHz. Such a small variation agrees with our attribution of the process to the surfactant exchange between the water phase and the interfacial film. Indeed the same surfactant (SDS) was used throughout this work and its exchange kinetics should not be too affected by the type of oil.

Finally, it should be noticed that measurements performed on a microemulsion system containing a surfactant with a very long alkyl chain may prove much easier to interpret. Indeed this surfactant would exchange very slowly[13] and if the corresponding relaxation is well below 1MHz, the relaxational excess absorption for such systems in the 1-155MHz range should be characterized by a single relaxation frequency associated with the alcohol exchange. Such possibility is currently being considered.

3) Attempt of Interpretation of the Changes of the Relaxation Parameters with Composition

The complexity of microemulsions from both purely chemical and structural points of views makes it difficult to go beyond a qualitative interpretation of the characteristics of the two exchange processes. For the reasons which will appear below we first consider System I.

The decrease of f_{R1} and f_{R2} in the O/W range, upon addition of cyclohexane can be understood on the basis of Aniansson's[13,24] expression for the relation frequency for the exchange process

$$2 \pi f_R = \frac{k^-}{n} \ \frac{C_M}{C} + \frac{k^-}{\sigma^2} \qquad \qquad \ldots (3)$$

n is the number of exchanging species per aggregate, σ is the standard deviation of n (σ increases with n), k^- is the rate constant for the dissociation of one exchanging species from the aggregate and C and C_M are the concentrations of the free and aggregated species. In using equation 3 for the surfactant exchange the coupling between the two exchange processes[25] has been neglected. However, this approximation is not unreasonable for the type of qualitative interpretation which is sought here. It is also understood that equation 3 can be used with systems as complicated as microemulsions only for such purpose.

Upon addition of oil to a water/surfactant/alcohol system, n and thus σ are increased[26] and the concentration C of free exchanging species is decreased[20]. As $C \approx k^-/k^+$ where k^+ is the diffusion controlled association rate constant of an exchanging species to an aggregate[5,13], k^- is also decreased. Thus f_R should progressively be decreased upon addition of oil. This prediction holds for both the surfactant and alcohol. Since the relaxation amplitude is proportional to f_R^{-1}, A will increase as the oil content is increased. Thus the straightforward extension of an equation valid for micellar solutions to O/W microemulsions provides an explanation of their ultrasonic relaxation behaviour upon increasing oil content.

In W/O microemulsions the above equation may hold for the alcohol exchange between the interfacial layer and the oil phase. This equation is however more difficult to handle since the relative changes of n, C_M and k^- cannot be simply assessed. The equation 3 does not hold for the surfactant exchange. For this process, however, a simple reasoning leads to the conclusion that f_{R1} is independent of the water volume fraction ψ_w whereas A_1 is proportional to ψ_w if the composition of the interfacial layer and the concentration of surfactant in the aqueous phase remain constant upon addition of oil. Of the three investigated Systems, System I is the one where these conditions are the most closely met. Indeed, the representative points of the seven investigated solutions fall close to a straight line originating from the oil apex. This means that the (alcohol)/ (SDS) is almost constant, and in turn that the composition of the interfacial film is also nearly constant. The results in Fig. 3 show that in fact f_{R1} increases slightly with the oil content. This may reflect a small change of the surfactant concentration in the water core. In any case, for the W/O range equation 2 explains the decrease of A_1 upon increasing oil content.

The above discussion thus leads to predict an increase of the relaxation amplitude with the oil content in the O/W range and a decrease in the W/O range, and thus the presence of a maximum in the intermediate range, that is the transition range. It is however noteworthy pointing out that in the transition range the change of f_{R1} and f_{R2} is very progressive. This is in fact a fairly general feature of our results which suggests for microemulsions some kind of bicontinuous structure, which could be similar to the ones postulated by Scriven[28]. Bicontinuous structures have also been invoked to explain the progressive change of diffusion coefficient of various microemulsion components upon composition changes[29].

This type of reasoning presented above cannot be used to try to explain the results for Systems IIa and III because in the conditions

where the experiments were performed all the characteristics of these
Systems are modified (number and radius of the particles, composition
of the continuous phases). However equation 2 still holds and predicts
a continuous decrease of A_1 in the W/O range, in agreement with the
experimental results. When the work reported in Part I was performed
the W/O to O/W transition range was believed to be located on the
demixing line of the System IIa phase diagram for almost equal weight
percents of toluene and water. Since then new investigations by means
of quasi elastic light scattering have suggested that this range is
rather close to the water apex[27]. Thus, the extension of the W/O
range would be much larger than previously reported. The same behaviour is expected for System III. These new results may explain why
the results of Figs.7,9 and 14 show a monotonous decrease of A_1 in
such a large range of oil content. For these Systems measurements
performed at a different (alcohol)/(SDS) ratio and with compositions
having representative points falling on a line originating from the
toluene or dodecane apex would probably reveal a relaxation behaviour
similar to that of System I provided that the investigated compositions include the transition range.

CONCLUSIONS

    The results reported in this study confirm and extend those
obtained previously. The ultrasonic relaxation investigations of some
thirty microemulsions pertaining to three different quaternary systems
did not reveal any ultrasonic absorption effect which could be related
to critical phenomena. The ultrasonic absorption of O/W as well as
W/O microemulsions has been found to be generally characterized by
two relaxation processes. The slow process has been attributed to the
exchange of the surfactant between the interfacial film and the aqueous phase (whether continuous or dispersed) whereas the fast process
was assigned to the exchange of the alcohol between the interfacial
film and the aqueous and oil phases. Some of the characteristics of
the relaxation processes can be qualitatively explained by extending
an equation valid for micellar solutions. The most puzzling feature
of the data is probably the very continuous change of the relaxation
parameters with composition even in the range where W/O microemulsions
turn into O/W microemulsions. Such a result lends support to the
assumption of a bicontinuous structure for the compositions in this
range.

ACKNOWLEDGEMENT

    The authors thank the DGRST (France) for its financial support
(Grant 77.7.1456).

REFERENCES

1. J. Lang, A. Djavanbakht and R. Zana, J. Phys. Chem., 84, 1541
    (1980).

2.   A. Skoulios and D. Guillon, J. Phys. Lett., 38, L-137 (1977).

3.   M. Dvolaitzky. M. Guyot, M. Laguës, J.-P. Le Pesant, R. Ober,
     C. Sauterey and C. Taupin, J. Chem. Phys., 69, 3279 (1978).

4.   M. Laguës, R. Ober and C. Taupin, J. Phys. Lett., 39, L-487
     (1978).

5.   S. Yiv and R. Zana, J. Colloid Interface Sci., 65, 286, (1978);
     S. Yiv, R. Zana, W. Ulbricht and H. Hoffmann, J. Colloid Inter-
     face Sci., 80, 224 (1981).

6.   A. Djavanbakht, J. Lang and R. Zana, J. Phys. Chem., 81, 2620
     and 2630, (1977).

7.   M. Dinh-Cao and J. Lang, to be published

8.   M. Fixman, J. Chem. Phys., 36, 1961, (1962).

9.   M. Breazeale, J. Chem. Phys., 36, 2530, (1962); E. Bains and
     M. Breazeale, J. Chem. Phys., 61, 1238 (1974); Ibid., 62, 742
     (1975).

10. A. Anantaraman, A. Walters, P. Edmonds and C. Pings, J. Chem.
     Phys., 44, 2651 (1966).

11. G. D'Arrigo and D. Sette, J. Chem. Phys., 48, 691 (1968).

12. E. Graber, J. Lang and R. Zana, Kolloid Z.Z. Polym., 237, 470
     (1970).

13. E. Aniansson, S. Wall, M. Almgren, H. Hoffmann, I. Kielmann,
     W. Ulbricht, R. Zana, J. Lang and C. Tondre, J. Phys. Chem.,
     80, 905 (1976).

14. M. J. Blandamer, N. Hidden, M. Symons and N. Treloar, Trans.
     Faraday Soc., 64, 3242 (1968).

15. K. Tamura, M. Maekawa and T. Yasunaga, J. Phys. Chem., 81, 2122
     (1977).

16. S. Nishikawa, M. Mashima and T. Yasunaga, Bull. Chem. Soc. Jap.
     50, 3047 (1977) and references therein.

17. A. Graciaa, J. Lachaise, A. Martinez, M. Bourrel and C. Chambu
     C. R. Hebd. Séan. Acad. Sci., B 282, 547 (1976).

18. G. Goset, Ph.D. Thesis, Université de Pau et des Pays de l'Adour,
     Académie de Bordeaux, (1978).

19. M. Eigen and L. De Maeyer "Investigation of Rates and Mechanisms
     of Reactions" in "Technique of Organic Chemistry" S. Friess,
     E. Lewis, A. Weissberger, Ed., Interscience: New York, 1959,
     vol. VIII, Part II.

20. K. Hayase and S. Hayano, Bull. Chem. Soc. Jap., 50 83 (1977);
     N. Singh and S. Swarup, Bull. Chem. Soc. Jap., 51 1534 (1978).

21. A. M. Cazabat, D. Langevin and A. Pouchelon, J. Colloid Inter-
     face Sci., 73, 1 (1980), and references therein.

22. This volume change is assumed to be equal to that for the
     exchange of the surfactant between the micelles and the bulk
     solution in micellar solutions.

23. J. Corkill, J. Goodman and T. Walker, Trans. Faraday Soc., 63,
     768 (1967); S. Kaneshima, M. Tanaka, T. Tomida and R. Matuura,
     J. Colloid Interface Sci., 48, 450 (1974).

24. E. A. G. Aniansson and S. Wall, J. Phys. Chem., 79, 857 (1975).

25. E. A. G. Aniansson, "Techniques and Applications of Fast Reac-
     tions in Solutions", W. J. Gettins and E. Wyn-Jones Ed.,

         D. Reidel Publ. Co., 1979, p. 249.
26.   The number of surfactant molecules per microemulsion droplet
      is always much larger than that of pure surfactant micelles.
      See for instance ref. 3.
27.   A. Bellocq and G. Fourche, J. Colloid Interface Sci., 78, 275 (1980)
28.   L. E. Scriven, "Micellization, Solubilization and Microemul-
      sions" K. L. Mittal Ed., Plenum Press, 1977, Vol. II, p. 877.
29.   F. Larche, J. Rouriere, P. Delord, B. Brun and J. Dussossoy,
      J. Phys. Lett., 41, L-437 (1980).

DISCUSSION

Prof. B. Lemanceau: Are there lamellar phases in these systems?

Dr. J. Lang: The possibility of the existence of lamellar structures
in the System made of water/SDS/1-butanol/toluene has been put forward
by P. Lalanne et al. (C. R. Hebd. Séan. Acad. Sci., C 286, 55 (1978)
and J. Chim. Phys., 75, 236 (1978) on the basis of viscosity, NMR and
electron microscopy experiments. From our experimental results,
however, it is not possible to tell if lamellar phases are present.

Dr. W. Knoche: Is it possible that there are contributions from more
than two relaxation processes?

Dr. J. Lang: In the case of ternary systems composed of water,
surfactant and alcohol it is known that three relaxation processes
exist in some cases as for instance with tetradecyltrimethylammonium
bromide and 1-pentanol: the two faster processes are due to the
exchange of the surfactant and of the alcohol molecules between the
mixed micelles and the water-rich continuous phase, the slow process
being due to the complete dissolution or formation of the micelle.
Thus, along the water-(SDS + 1-butanol) axis of the phase diagram of
the water/SDS/1-butanol/toluene system (see Fig. 5) and for a high
content of water, three relaxation processes are present. However
the slow process is not detectable by the ultrasonic absorption
technique used in this work. I am not aware of experimental results
obtained for the slow relaxation process for high concentrations of
SDS + 1-butanol in water (corresponding to point S11 in Fig. 5 for
instance). I am not aware either of experimental work done on the
slow process in case of quaternary or pseudoternary systems. I would
guess however that if oil is added the slow relaxation process would
be characterized by a long relaxation time and will perhaps not be
detectable by a usual relaxation technique. Other possible relaxation
processes, which could appear in the ultrasonic absorption frequencies
domain, have been discussed in the paper and shown to have negligible
contributions.

Dr. M. McDonald: For the system octanoate-butanol-water where there
two relaxation processes and how did you interpret?

Dr. J. Lang: No ultrasonic absorption spectra have been made on the sodium octanoate/1-butanol/water system which has been only studied at 3.65 MHz. However, spectroscopic measurements on some ternary systems made of surfactant, alcohol and water have shown the existence of two relaxation processes which have been attributed to the exchange of the surfactant and of the alcohol molecules between the mixed micelles and the water-rich continuous phase. Two relaxation processes have been for instance obtained in the present work for ternary systems made of SDS, 1-butanol or 1-pentanol and water.

Prof. F. Franks: I am intrigued by the complete absence of concentration fluctuations near the demixing lines in ternary systems. Does this not imply that the phase transition is 100% cooperative?

Dr. J. Lang: We have shown that for ternary systems (sodium octanoate/1-butanol/water, n-hexane/2-propanol/water) the ultrasonic absorption technique is sensitive to concentration fluctuations near the demixing lines, these fluctuations being smaller than in the case of binary systems. On the contrary for the pseudoternary systems studied in our work, the ultrasonic absorption measurements have not revealed the existence of concentration fluctuations neither near demixing lines nor in composition regions where transitions of W/O to O/W structures are known to occur. The question then arises if the phase transition is not 100% cooperative in the case of pseudoternary systems. Numerous measurements have been made for compositions very close to the demixing lines and none of them have shown a large increase of the absorption which could have been attributed to concentration fluctuations. Furthermore in case of the water/SDS/1-butanol/toluene system the measurements made along line DC (see Fig. 7 in reference 1) have been pursued even for compositions in the polyphasic domain, just after demixing. The values of the absorption were about the same as those found in the monophasic domain around the representative point C.

Aerosol OT, 18, 33, 38, 221
Alcohol, fluorinated, 94
Ammonium sulphate, 11
Amphiphile, 115, 116
t-Amyl alcohol, 68
Anisotropic motion, 154, 158
Antonov's rule, 142
Auto-correlation function, 35, 36
Benzene, 9, 88
Benzyl alcohol, 7
Bicontinuous
  interspersion, 68, 79
  microemulsion, 77
  state, 19, 114, 117, 251
Bimolecular reactions, 174
Birefringence
  optical, 52, 186
  streaming, 111
Bragg spacing, 52
Brine, 65, 131
i-Butyl alcohol 68, 233

Chemical shift, 23
Chloroform, 88
Clausius-Clapeyron equation, 194
Clipped correlation technique, 37
Cloud point, 5, 95
Coexistence curve, 194
Collision
  densities, 174
  rate, 44
  sticky, 44, 217, 230

Conductivity, 28, 66, 147, 207
Copolymers, 49
Correlation time, 27
Cosurfactant, 30, 55, 115
Counterion, 117, 149
Cyclohexane, 1, 40
Cylides de Dupin, 59

Demixing line, 240, 255
Dielectric dispersion, 103
Di-2-ethylhexyl sulfosuccinates, 19
Diffusion
  coefficient, 19, 35, 41, 116, 210
  self, 115, 117, 122, 125
Di-palmitoyl-phosphatidyl choline, 185
Dodecyl trimethylammonium chloride, 117
Dynamic light scattering, 33

Entropy of mixing, 112
Ethyl alcohol, 9

Fast-freeze, 160
Floc, 156
Fluorescer, 224
Fluorocarbons, 86
Focal conic
  parabolic, 59
  textures, 59
Friction coefficient, 36, 42

Gibbs distribution function, 177
Gibbs phase triangle, 3

Half line-width, 25, 159
Hamiltonian, 174, 177
Hanai equation, 108
n-Heptane, 40
Hexanol, 108
HLB, 4, 88, 92
Hofmeister series, 15
Hydrodynamic radii, 20, 39
Hydrogen bridge, 21

Intensity autocorrelation
    function, 19, 38
Interfacial tension, 2, 6, 46,
        131, 138
Inverse cylindrical structure, 62
Isopiestic vapour sorption, 146
Isothermal compressibility, 28

Kerr-effect, 25
Kink-step, 197

Laser-temperature-jumper, 187
Lennard-Jones potential, 174
Liposomes, 185
Liquid-crystal, 57, 160
    cubic, 116, 120
    hexagonal, 120
    lamellar, 19, 28, 111, 116
Low angle neutron scattering,
        40, 164

Method of cumulants, 38
Micelles
    inverse, 33, 62, 68
    oil swollen, 66
    rod, 83, 170
    reversed, 103, 104, 119, 222,
        229
    spherical, 76, 222
Miscibility gap, 3, 4
Moire patterns, 160
Myeline-structures, 186

Nonylphenylether, 1

i-Octane, 7, 40, 223
Onsager equation, 151
Opacity, 70
Order parameters, 123, 201
Osmotic-compressibility, 42

Pair-correlation function, 179,
        184
Partition coefficient, 56
Pentan-1-ol, 33, 131, 210, 233
Percolation, 68, 217
    threshold, 77, 78
Permittivity, 104, 106
    complex 113
Phase-inversion, 1, 91, 104
Phase-smectic, 59
Phospholipid, 185
Photon correlation spectroscopy,
        37
Polarizability, 30, 35
Polydispersity, 19, 38, 83
Polyhedra, Voronoi, 76
Polystyrene sulphonate, 21
Pressure-jump, 188
Pseudo-quaternary system, 11
Pseudo-ternary phase diagram, 53,
        132
Pulsed-gradient spin-echo, 125

Quasi-elastic light scattering, 19

Radius of gyration, 100, 166
Random coil, 100
Refractive index, 138

Salinity, 65, 135
Scattering
    function, 36
    multiple, 46
    neutron intensity, 88, 100, 233
    wave vector, 35
    x-ray, 99, 145
Smectic phase, 170
Sodium cetyl sulfate, 213
Sodium cholate, 122
Sodium dodecyl sulfate, 33, 118,
        152, 233
Sodium 4-(1-heptyl nonyl) benzene
        sulfonate, 68, 144
Sodium octanoate, 118
Sodium octylbenzene sulfonate,
        120, 131
Solubility parameter, 90
Spherulitic particles, 145
Spinning drop method, 131
    tensiometer, 142

Spin-spin relaxation time, 25
Stokes-Einstein equation, 42,
      213, 218
Stopped-flow technique, 229
Structure factor, 36
Surface tension, 90
Surfactants
   double tail, 143, 167
   fluorinated, 86, 90
   polymeric, 49

Tertiary oil recovery, 11, 131
Tetraoxyethylene glycol dodecyl
   ether, 104, 122
Tie-lines, 3, 4, 135, 136
Toluene, 40, 50
Triton X-100, 89, 108
Turbidity, 197
   point, 131, 144
Tween 40, 60,   209

Ultracentrifuge, 23
Ultrasonic
   absorption, 197, 234, 243
   relaxation, 233
Upper critical temperature, 4
Upper phase boundary, 28

Vesicles, 170, 185, 189
Viscometer
   multiphase rolling ball, 69
   Ostwald, 208
Viscosity, 27, 66, 117, 214

Walden's rule, 208
Water 'pools', 111, 113, 205,
      229

X-ray diffraction, 52, 117, 164